HIV-1 and Communication Disorders

What Speech and Hearing Professionals Need to Know

HIV-1 and Communication Disorders

What Speech and Hearing Professionals Need to Know

Connie R. Larsen, M.S., CCC-SLP

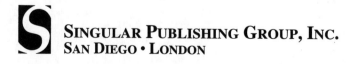
SINGULAR PUBLISHING GROUP, INC.
SAN DIEGO • LONDON

Singular Publishing Group, Inc.
401 West "A" Street, Suite 325
San Diego, California 92101-7904

Singular Publishing Ltd.
19 Compton Terrace
London N1 2UN, UK

Singular Publishing Group, Inc., publishes textbooks, clinical manuals, clinical reference books, journals, videos, and multimedia materials on speech-language pathology, audiology, otorhinolaryngology, special education, early childhood, aging, occupational therapy, physical therapy, rehabilitation, counseling, mental health, and voice. For your convenience, our entire catalog can be accessed on our website at **http://www.singpub.com**. Our mission to provide you with materials to meet the daily challenges of the ever-changing health care/educational environment will remain on course if we are in touch with you. In that spirit, we welcome your feedback on our products. Please telephone **(1-800-521-8545)**, fax **(1-800-774-8398)**, or e-mail **(singpub@mail.cerfnet.com**) your comments and requests to us.

©1998 by Singular Publishing Group, Inc.

Typeset in 10/12 Palatino Light by Thompson Type
Printed in the United States of America by McNaughton & Gunn

Library of Congress Cataloging-in-Publication Data

Larsen, Connie R.
    HIV-1 and communication disorders : what speech and hearing
professionals need to know / by Connie R. Larsen.
        p.   cm. — (Singular textbook series)
    Includes bibliographical references and index.
    ISBN 1-56593-968-9
        1. Communicative disorders.   2. AIDS (Disease)—Complications.
3. Neurologic manifestations of general diseases.   4. Otologic
manifestations of general diseases.   5. Otologic manifestations of
general diseases.   I. Title.   II. Series.
RC423.L34   1998
616.85'5—DC21   98-3471
                                                                          CIP

Contents

7 Counseling Issues

Foreword

In the ever-expanding medical speech-language pathology field, HIV-1 and AIDS-related disorders that affect communication have only recently received research attention. Although the basic and applied medical research on HIV-1 infection and AIDS is extensive, relatively little has been written to help speech-language pathologists do their part in the clinical management of patients with AIDS. There has been a great need for a single, comprehensive source for speech-language pathologists to gain an understanding of one of the most dreaded diseases of the 20th century. Connie Larsen has fulfilled this need. She has ably accomplished the challenging task of summarizing what was until recently the most puzzling disease with a complex physiological mechanism producing varied and deadly consequences.

I am most impressed and pleased with this book not only because it fulfills a great need but also because how it does what it does. Readers of this book will note Connie's unstated compassion for people with AIDS subtly blended with her professional objectivity and unassuming scholarship. There is a finely woven but keenly felt sense of humility in this book. During the course of her writing, Connie repeatedly told me that there is not much research on communication assessment and treatment in patients with AIDS. She could not pretend to be an expert who can give advice to speech-language pathologists, she said. All she had done was to write a thesis on the subject, she often reminded me. Nonetheless, as the book shows, Connie has had a great deal to offer the profession.

Readers will recognize this as a groundbreaking attempt. I trust that this pioneering text and clinical resource book will be a part of expanding curriculum in medical speech-language pathology and clinical work in varied professional settings. I also trust that this leading work will stimulate more research and writing on the central nervous system disorders and resulting communicative impairments associated with AIDS. I know that Connie will be pleased if the book helps even a few speech-language pathologists understand HIV-1 infection a bit better and leads them to think that they can do a bit more for their patients with AIDS.

M. N. Hegde, Ph.D.
Singular Textbook Series Editor

Acknowledgments

During my senior year in college, one of my family members was diagnosed with acquired immunodeficiency syndrome (AIDS). David's illness progressed rapidly, and at one point, he received dysphagia therapy from a speech-language pathologist. This piqued my interest in how speech-language pathology services were being utilized in the management of AIDS-related communication disorders and dysphagia. As I sought answers to that question, the lack of information in the literature of speech-language pathology became very evident. During graduate school, I gathered research to answer my questions about the disease and the role of communication disorder specialists in AIDS management, and a passion grew for the subject. I wanted to share what I was learning with other professionals in the field of communication disorders. I wish to thank Singular Publishing Group for allowing me the opportunity to share through the publication of this book.

My special thanks to M. N. (Giri) Hegde, Ph.D., who spent many hours reading and editing the manuscript. His skill as an editor makes me appear to be a better writer than I am.

The influence of Carla Hess, Ph.D., permeates the contents of this book. Dr. Hess has been an inspiration and encouragement to me during my undergraduate and graduate years at the University of North Dakota and beyond. She has left a lasting imprint on my mind by being an excellent role-model as a scholar, a clinician, and a woman of integrity.

This book is dedicated to the memory of L. David Larsen, who died of AIDS on April 22, 1995.

Introduction

$\mathbf{A}$cquired immunodeficiency syndrome (AIDS) is one of the most feared and rapidly spreading diseases of the 20th century. In the last decade and a half, it has reached worldwide epidemic proportions. Worldwide, the statistics are startling. There are an estimated 8,500 new HIV-1 infections each day (1000 of them are children), 90% of cases occur in developing countries, 40% occur among women, and more than 50% of cases occur in persons between the ages of 15 and 25 years of age (Piot, 1997). It is projected that by the year 2000, between 30 and 40 million men, women, and children around the world will be infected with the human immunodeficiency virus type 1 (HIV-1), which causes AIDS (World Health Organization, 1992). Other sources have estimated that this number may be as high as 110 million (Mann, Tarantola, & Netter, 1992).

Scientists currently disagree about whether or not the AIDS epidemic has crested in the United States, but all are certain that many more children, teens, and adults will suffer tragically. By the turn of the century, AIDS will be the third most common cause of death in the United States. However, there have been many research advances in the last decade. Prophylactic interventions are reducing the incidence of the often lethal opportunistic infections, including *Pneumocystis carinii pneumonia* (Collier et al., 1996; Creagh-Kirk et al., 1988; Fischl et al., 1987). Persons with HIV-1 infection who have access to new life-prolonging drug therapies are living longer (Centers for Disease Control [CDC], 1992a). However, the longer life span increases concerns about the quality of life and productivity of those individuals.

Although education about AIDS is spreading faster than the disease itself, and the ways to avoid infection are well known, AIDS continues to be one of the world's greatest health problems. A substantial number of HIV-1-infected patients experience long-term disabilities involving cognitive and motor functions, which includes communication disorders (Flower & Sooy, 1987; Price et al., 1988; Sahakian et al., 1995; Watkins et al.,

1

1990). Neurological symptoms are present in 40 to 60% of all AIDS patients, and central nervous system (CNS) involvement represents the principle cause of death in that population (Gray, Hurtrel, & Hurtrel, 1993; Meyaard, Otto, Keet, Ross, & Miedema, 1992). Neuropathological studies by autopsy have demonstrated that nearly 100% of patients with AIDS have pathological abnormalities in the CNS (Ciardi, Sinclair, Scaravilli, Harcout-Webster, & Lucas, 1990; Gray et al., 1993; Neuen-Jacob, Arendt, von Giesen, & Wechsler, 1996).

The high incidence rates for CNS lesions documented in HIV-1-infected patients indicate that these patients would have associated secondary speech and language disorders, hearing impairment, cognitive deficits, and dysphagia. There should be speech-language pathologists in medical settings who currently have persons with AIDS on their caseload. In large urban areas, speech-language pathologists employed in the school setting would have pediatric cases of AIDS on their caseloads. However, a review of the literature in speech-language pathology (SLP) revealed a paucity of information pertaining to HIV and AIDS. In speech-language pathology, there is limited information on the history of the disease, the nature of the virus, incidence rates, sites of lesion, or case management.

This paucity of information was the motivation for researching and writing *Associated Communication Disorders and Dysphagia in Adults with HIV-1 and Secondary CNS Lesions* (Larsen, 1996) for the completion of my master's degree. Because this book is based largely on my study, I have provided a brief description of the research method used in my original study.

The extensive review of the literature undertaken to complete this study revealed that no one discipline contained all the necessary data for an accurate clinical profile. Each of the different disciplines had essential data components of the profile. Therefore, the profile of the adult with HIV-1and CNS lesions with associated communication disorders and dysphagia was generated by synthesizing the numerical and narrative data found in the fields of biological sciences, medicine, neuropathology, psychology, and speech-language pathology. Content analysis, one of many qualitative methods of organizing and analyzing data, was used in the study.

The qualitative research paradigm has its roots in cultural anthropology and American sociology (Kirk & Miller, 1986). Educational researchers only recently have adopted qualitative research methods (Borg & Gall, 1989; Gay, 1996). The intent of qualitative research is to understand a particular phenomenon, event, role, group, or interaction. In this type of research, the researcher gradually makes sense out of a phenomenon of interest by contrasting, comparing, replicating, cataloging, and classifying the object under study (Miles & Huberman, 1984). The researcher looks for categories, patterns, and themes that will facilitate a coherent synthesis of available data. This synthesis represents the researcher's overall understanding of what the data mean.

Traditional quantitative research designs may better be applied after careful qualitative analyses have identified most of the relevant variables. Especially troublesome is the potential for misinterpretation due to confounding factors. For example, individuals who experience pain or discomfort in the speech mechanism may use compensatory movements to reduce discomfort in speech and this could generate abnormal speech characteristics. The researcher may incorrectly judge the individual's compensatory speech behavior to be due to CNS involvement.

In quantitative measurement, validity is the degree to which an instrument measures what it intends to measure. Reliability is the consistency with which the same phenomenon is measured. When standardized instruments are used, reliability and validity refer to the measures themselves.

On the other hand, in qualitative research, the concepts of validity and reliability still are relevant but must be considered differently than in quantitative research. In qualitative research, the researcher is the de facto instrument, or the only instrument for data collection. Thus, the quality of data is based on the quality of the instrument (the researcher). This suggests one of the criticisms associated with qualitative research, namely, the inability to adequately assess the validity and reliability of data due to inherent biases of the researcher. A common strategy designed to address these biases is *triangulation.*

Triangulation is the act of bringing multiple sources of data together to corroborate, elaborate, or illuminate the phenomena under study (Marshall & Rossman, 1995). The purpose of triangulation is to seek convergence of results. Derived from navigation science, triangulation has been applied to social science research to enhance the external validity of a study. Therefore, in my study, I used the process of triangulation to generate data, resulting in the clinical profile of a client with HIV-1 infection.

Designing a study in which multiple cases or data-gathering methods are utilized can greatly strengthen the study's applicability for other settings. The process of triangulation in my study involved the use of data from various disciplines. Each field has a different research focus on HIV-1 and reports information from the perspective of its own professional concerns. In this study, the perspectives of five fields of research yielded multiple associated foci:

- medicine: sites of lesions, incidence data, clinical manifestations and pathologies, and medical management of symptoms
- neuropathology and neurobiology: autopsy data regarding neural pathogenesis, sites of lesion, and incidence

- general science: cellular and molecular biology, physiology, and pathology
- psychiatry/psychology: cognitive behavioral manifestations
- speech-language pathology and audiology: identification and management of speech, language, and hearing disorders and dysphagia

When the content analysis was completed, all the necessary data needed to generate the target profile was in place. The completed clinical profile was the interpretation of that data. The data generated for the above study (Larsen, 1996) provides the clinical framework for this book.

The writing of this book was undertaken for the primary purpose of educating speech-language pathologists and audiologists in how HIV-1 infection and AIDS affect communication sciences and disorders. This book serves as an introduction to core concepts about the disease and its implications for speech-language pathology and audiology. It also is written to encourage future research in the area of HIV-1-related communication disorders. Much information is presented in this book, but there are multiple questions left unanswered. It is hoped that the information presented here will trigger a desire within communication disorders specialists to find answers to those many questions.

Chapter 1 provides a succinct review of the history and current status of HIV-1 and AIDS in the United States. This information is a synthesis of data obtained from an extensive review of literature in medicine, neuropathology, cellular and molecular biology, physiology, communication disorders, and government agencies concerned with AIDS and HIV-1. As the history is reviewed, core concepts about HIV-1 are introduced.

Chapter 2 is a discussion about the effects of HIV-1 infection on the body and stages of disease progression. Information on pathologies and conditions that could affect speech, language, cognition, swallow function, and hearing during each phase of infection is described.

Chapters 3, 4, and 5 provide clinical information on communication disorders associated with adult HIV-1-infection. Chapter 3 is an overview of clinical management, with a section of the chapter providing information on occupational exposure to HIV-1. Chapter 4 discusses central nervous system manifestations associated with HIV-1 infection. Chapter 5 presents information on the head and neck manifestations, otologic findings, and information on dysphagia and odynophagia related to HIV-1 infection.

Pediatric HIV-1 infection and the related issues are presented in Chapter 6. There are special concerns in this population, and the course and severity of the disease frequently is altered in children.

Chapter 7 discusses the sensitive topic of counseling when working with clients with HIV-1 infection and AIDS. Even in the best of environments, facing death at an early age while suffering from one infection after another would be devastating. For many people with AIDS, there is no support network. This chapter provides resources to refer clients and significant others to a variety of sources of help and information.

These data were compiled to introduce speech-language pathologists and audiologists to clinical and behavioral symptoms that could be expected in clients with HIV-1 infection. Education in the phases of HIV-1 infection and the associated communication disorders may help the professional determine if new deficits that may arise are due to disease progression or secondary to medications in use. In addition, accurate information is provided regarding the risk to the clinician of working with patients who have HIV-1.

It is hoped that the data presented in this book will provide the bases for much-needed research in the field of communication disorders. There is need for efficacy data regarding the success of using traditional therapy methods with persons with HIV-1 infection. The reporting of individual case studies would be beneficial.

In addition to communication disorders professionals, this book may serve as a reference for special educators, for caregivers who work with persons with HIV-1 infection, and for those who have HIV-1 infection. It is hoped that the information presented in this book may provide insight into how to communicate more effectively with individuals who live with HIV-1 infection.

1

History of HIV-1 in the United States

The year 1981 frequently is cited as the start of the AIDS epidemic, but HIV-1 is not a new virus. In 1952, a physician in Manchester, England, had a patient who died a mysterious death. The physician froze a specimen of the man's blood in hopes that in the future, medical knowledge would be able to determine what caused this type of illness and death. The use of a sophisticated technique known as polymerase chain reaction conclusively confirmed that this man did in fact have AIDS. Although the virus did exist for decades, it did not begin to take the devastating toll on humankind until 1981. It was in 1981 that medical professionals became aware of unusual cases of otherwise healthy young men being diagnosed with rare diseases.

HIV-1 AND AIDS IN THE UNITED STATES FROM 1981–1997

First Reported Cases of AIDS

On June 5, 1981, the Centers for Disease Control (CDC, 1981a) reported in *Morbidity and Mortality Weekly Report (MMWR)* about five individuals who presented with an unusual form of pneumonia caused by a parasite called *Pneumocystis carinii*. On July 4, 1981, Kaposi's sarcoma, which previously had been an uncommonly reported skin malignancy in the United States, was diagnosed in 26 homosexual men in both New York City and California (CDC, 1981b). In August 1981, it was noted, that in addition to *Pneumocystis carinii* and Kaposi's sarcoma, a variety of other opportunistic diseases were being reported in homosexual men (CDC, 1981c).

In May 1982, the occurrence of persistent and generalized lymphadenopathy, or enlarged lymph nodes, was being reported among homosexual men in Atlanta, New York, and San Francisco (CDC, 1982a). Approximately 70% of these patients had other symptoms, including fatigue, fever, night sweats, and weight loss of at least five pounds. Although many individuals reported a history of other sexually-transmitted infections, such as gonorrhea, syphilis, and amebiases, none of these infections adequately explained the occurrence of lymphadenopathy. Studies of these cases revealed very low levels of **T-helper lymphocyte** in these patients (CDC, 1982b). T-helper lymphocytes are an important part of the human immune system.

All living organisms are constantly exposed to **pathogens** (substances that are capable of causing harm). Most organisms have protective mechanisms such as physical barriers (e.g., blood-brain barrier) in place or chemicals that repel or kill invading organisms or foreign substances. Humans have complex immune systems. The human immune system is a complex network of organs containing cells that recognize and destroy pathogens. Specific parts of the immune system include **phagocytes** that destroy and eat foreign substances and cells, **natural killer cells** that attack cancer cells, **cytotoxic T-cells** that circulate throughout the body to identify viral antigens on the surfaces of cells, and **B-cells** that are able to change into a plasma cell that produces antibodies that disable viral antigens. Research revealed that the human immune system was particularly vulnerable to the new virus.

Viruses are not living creatures and are dependent on host cells to carry out metabolic functions such as reproduction. A virus is a piece of nucleic acid with a protein coating. Viruses may be composed of either ribonucleic acid (RNA) or deoxyribonucleic acid (DNA) proteins, but not both. HIV-1 is a **retrovirus**, which means it is composed of RNA proteins. With a special enzyme (a catalyst) called **reverse transcriptase**, a retrovirus can produce an analog, or copy, of itself. This copy is a DNA form of the virus that implants itself into the genetic material of the host cell. Once the genetic material is commanded by the virus, the cell follows the DNA program of the virus, which transforms the host cell into a virus-producing factory. A descriptive analogy of this relationship is that of a computer disk (software) in relation to a computer (hardware). Necessary metabolic functions required to support the host cell are interrupted by the viral program and the virus eventually kills the host cell, depleting essential cells of the immune system.

Once the virus gains access into target cells within the immune system, the virus is effectively concealed from the other immune cells that circulate throughout the body searching for foreign substances. Host cells in the immune system are not only used to produce more HIV-1, but also as Trojan horses that conceal the virus from the defense mechanism of the body.

In September 1982, the term **acquired immune deficiency syndrome** (AIDS) was introduced (CDC, 1982c). The CDC proposed its first definition of AIDS as a "disease at least moderately predictive of a defect in cell-mediated immunity occurring in a person with no known cause for diminished resistance to that disease. Such diseases include Kaposi's sarcoma, *Pneumocystis carinii* pneumonia, and serious opportunistic infections." The CDC recognized that this definition did not include the full spectrum of AIDS manifestations.

In late 1982, the reports of Pneumocystis pneumonia in persons with hemophilia (a hereditary blood disease characterized by failure of blood to clot and abnormal bleeding to occur) raised the possibility of a blood-borne infectious agent, because these males were heterosexual and none had a history of intravenous drug abuse (CDC, 1982d). Medical experts in New York City, New Jersey, and San Francisco reported cases of AIDS in infants and young children (CDC, 1982e). The majority of these children were born to mothers who were at high risk for AIDS, and it was thought that transmission from mother to child in utero or shortly after birth could account for the early onset of immune deficiency.

AIDS Research in the Early 1980s

As research intensified, two groups of investigators emerged as leaders in AIDS research. One group was headed by Dr. Robert Gallo of the National Institutes of Health in Bethesda, Maryland. Dr. Luc Montagnier of the Pasteur Institute in Paris, France, led the second investigative group. In February 1983, Gallo proposed that AIDS was probably caused by a retrovirus. Retroviruses are characterized by the presence of a special enzyme, reverse transcriptase, which enables them to convert from an RNA to a DNA copy.

In May 1983, Montagnier's group published information in *Science* regarding the isolation of a retrovirus from an AIDS case with lymphadenopathy (Barre-Sinoussi et al., 1983). The virus was identified from the individual's lymph nodes and was, therefore, named the lymphadenopathy associated virus (LAV). In May 1984, Gallo's investigative group reported the same type of virus from two AIDS cases and named the virus HTLV-III (Gallo et al., 1984; Popovic, Sarngadharan, Read, & Gallo, 1984). HTLV stood for Human T-cell Lymphotrophic Virus, indicating the primary cell that the virus attacked. Type I and type II viruses had previously been associated with the development of leukemia in human beings. The U. S. Department of Health and Human Services officially assumed a double generic name for the virus, calling it HTLV-III/LAV in recognition of the contributions of both the American and French investigators.

The capacity of HTLV-III/LAV to cause immune suppression was well documented by December 1985 but new studies (Ho et al., 1985; Resnick et al., 1985) clarified that the virus could directly attack the central nervous system (CNS). These studies demonstrated that the virus was active within the CNS and was the most probable cause of a number of neurological syndromes seen among AIDS patients (Barnes, 1986; Schneider et al., 1983). The most common of these syndromes was a form of dementia. The studies isolated the HTLV-III/LAV from cerebrospinal fluid, and from brain, spinal cord, and peripheral nerve tissue of AIDS cases with various neurologic symptoms.

In May 1986, the International Committee on the Taxonomy of Viruses proposed to rename HTLV-III/LAV as the **human immunodeficiency virus** or HIV. Since that time, the term HIV has been used by the scientific community, media, and official organizations. The CDC (1986) proposed a new classification system for HIV-related infections in the same year. The classification system recognized the growing spectrum of HIV-related illness and offered a better means to group patients infected with HIV.

The CDC was able to publish the first set of statistics that signaled a slowing of the spread of HIV-1 infection at the end of 1986 (CDC, 1983, 1985). Although approximately 35,000 cases of AIDS had been reported in the United States, it was noted that the period of time required to double the number of cases was approximately thirteen months. This length of time was greater than the original estimation of six months as the doubling period that was reported early on in the epidemic.

AIDS Research in the Mid-1980s

Researchers at the CDC, led by Dr. Donald Francis, already were aware that there was a correlation between hepatitis and HIV-1: 80% of those with AIDS tested positive for hepatitis. Although the hepatitis screening tests were not specific in identifying HIV, it was the most accurate method available to remove infected blood from the blood supply at that time. Dr. Francis recommended that all blood banks test and subsequently destroy all blood that tested positive for hepatitis. Officials from the Red Cross and other blood banks argued that this was an alarmist reaction and decided not to screen for hepatitis as a possible marker for HIV-1-infected blood. Later, blood-screening tests in San Francisco and other metropolitan areas were to reveal that 1 in 500 people who received blood transfusions contracted the HIV-1 virus. It was not until 1986 that the federal government instituted a requirement that the blood bank industry test blood products for HIV-1 infection.

Major research findings occurred rapidly in 1984 and 1985. In October 1984, an investigative group cultured the virus from the semen of two homosexuals with AIDS in San Francisco, thus confirming the potential for the sexual transmission of the virus (Ho et al., 1984; Zagury et al., 1984). A major breakthrough occurred when several researchers established the molecular makeup of the HIV. In December of 1984, Shaw et al. (1984) reported their findings on the characterization of the structure of the virus. In 1985, the genetic makeup of the AIDS virus was established (Ratner et al., 1985; Wong-Staal et al., 1985). Research conducted by several laboratories confirmed that HIV-1 is a member of the lentivirus subfamily of human retroviruses. The characteristics the AIDS virus shares with lentiviruses include its long genome, highly variable envelope genes, induction of a slow disease, cytopathic (ability to injure or destroy a cell) properties in cell culture, and a tendency to infect the brain (Ho et al., 1985; Levy et al., 1985).

It was proposed that after fusing or binding with the cell membrane, HIV-1 enters the cell and injects its core into the cell. The core includes two identical strands of RNA. DNA polymerase makes a single-strand DNA copy of viral RNA, then a second DNA copy is made using the first as a template. This double-strand DNA is incorporated into the cell nucleus as a provirus and establishes a permanent infection. Much of the DNA of HIV-1 remains unintegrated in the cytoplasm. The HIV-1 replication cycle is restricted at this stage until the infected cell is activated. However, the activation process was not well understood at this time (Ho, Pomerantz, & Kaplan, 1987).

Scientists solved many of the puzzles about the genetic makeup of the HIV-1 in the mid- to late 1980s. The genome of HIV-1 was discovered to contain only three major genes: env, gag, and pol (Ratner et al., 1985). These genes were found to direct the formation of the basic components of HIV-1. The virus primarily infected cells with CD4 cell-surface receptor molecules, using them to gain entry into immune cells (Fahey et al., 1990; Klatzmann et al., 1984; Volberding et al., 1990). For entry of HIV-1 in macrophages and in some other cells lacking CD4 receptors, a complement receptor site was thought to be used instead. The primary targets of HIV-1 infection were demonstrated to be cells of the mononuclear phagocyte system, principally blood monocytes and tissue macrophages, T lymphocytes, B lymphocytes, natural killer lymphocytes, dendritic cells, Langerhans cells of epithelia and follicular cells in the brain, and gastrointestinal epithelial cells (Faulstich, 1986; Mehta & Kula, 1992).

Not all individuals who are exposed to HIV-1 become infected. Documentation about a small population of individuals who were **exposed but uninfected** (EU) began to appear in the literature. The probability of infection was hypothesized to be a function of several factors: the number of viruses (viral load) in the plasma or body fluid that a person is exposed to, genetic predisposition, route of exposure, and the number of cells available at the site of contact that have appropriate CD4 receptors (Burger, 1986).

HIV-1 was shown to have the additional ability to mutate easily. Due to the error rate of the reverse transcriptase enzyme, a mutation was introduced approximately once per 2000 incorporated nucleotides. This high mutation rate led to the emergence of HIV variants within the infected person's cells. These mutants could resist immune attack or drug therapy. They also could be more cytotoxic. Over time, different tissues of the body may harbor differing HIV variants. Therefore, the pattern of viral heterogeneity differs in different stages of disease (Pang et al., 1992).

There is an extended period before the development of any visible signs of infection. During this phase, there is little or no viral replication detectable in peripheral blood mononuclear cells and little or no culturable virus in peripheral blood. The CD4 lymphocyte count remains moderately decreased. However, the immune response to HIV-1 is insufficient to prevent continued viral replication within lymphoid tissues. Tests for HIV-1 antibody will remain positive during this time but antigen tests are usually negative.

Flower and Sooy (1987) published the first information regarding communication disorders associated with AIDS. The purpose of the article was to provide background information and to motivate speech-language pathologists and audiologists to fulfill the role of helping the AIDS patient communicate as long as possible. The article listed neurologic, ear, nose, and throat manifestations of AIDS that underlie communication disorders.

Increasing Public Awareness of AIDS

In the mid-1980s, the public still believed that AIDS was primarily a killer of gay men, even though officials knew that HIV was increasingly infecting hemophiliacs and those who had used contaminated needles for injection of illegal drugs. In 1985, the world learned that film star Rock Hudson suffered from AIDS. He became the first public figure known to have AIDS, and the public's ability to ignore AIDS began to crumble. Public dissatisfaction began to grow with the rate at which the government was providing information and research funding. Grassroots organizations formed by both gays and nongays emerged to deal with the growing AIDS crisis.

The gay-organized group that received the most media attention was AIDS Coalition to Unleash Power (ACT UP). This group used civil disobedience to call attention to federal government policies that the group believed needed to be changed. Primary issues were the Food and Drug Administration's (FDA) procedures that kept drugs in clinical trials for years and the lack of resources that were allocated to help prevent the spread of HIV. Many activists were frustrated at the lack of therapies available to those with HIV-1 infection. They expressed the belief that clinical trials of drugs that required long periods of time were pointless because the risk of taking a poorly researched therapy still had better odds for a cure compared to no treatment. The pressure on President Ronald Reagan and his administration to increase federal funding for public education on AIDS prevention and for AIDS research was growing.

In 1982, the first reports of pediatric AIDS appeared in the literature (CDC, 1982e). These reports found pediatric AIDS to occur in areas where there were high numbers of adult cases, specifically in families of AIDS patients. Initial reports suggested that children living in high-risk households were susceptible to AIDS. This news increased public fears that sexual contact, drug abuse, and exposure to contaminated blood products might not be the only ways of contracting the disease. (It was later found that perinatal transmission and hemophilia were the causes of these cases.) The initial public reaction was increased fear and hostility toward the HIV-1-positive population.

Some school systems prevented children with HIV-1 infection from participating in regular school activities. In the late 1980s, the plight of Ryan White, an adolescent who contracted HIV-1 infection through hemophilia and related blood transfusions, brought to public attention this heartbreaking situation. Ryan White became an advocate on behalf of other school-age children with AIDS and was invited to speak to Congress on the rights of these children. Due to the articulate and emotionally moving manner of this young man, the public became more enlightened and supportive of children infected with AIDS.

During the late 1980s, successful clinical trials of an antiretroviral drug known as AZT (3 azidothymidine) were reported by several researchers (Creagh-Kirk et al., 1988; Fischl et al., 1987; Marx, 1989). The studies demonstrated that AZT (also known as zidovudine and retrovir) was associated with a fourfold to sixfold reduction in the mortality rates in the study population at nine months. AZT, when used over a prolonged time period, decreased the incidence of opportunistic infections in AIDS patients as well as decreasing their overall mortality. These events prompted a rapid approval and deployment process for AZT. The use of **prophylactic** therapies (any agent or regimen that contributes to the prevention of infection and disease) enabled individuals with HIV infection to lead more productive lives because it allowed persons with chronic viral diseases to have periods of improvement between exacerbations.

In 1991, Earvin "Magic" Johnson, one of the country's greatest and best-loved professional basketball players, announced that he was infected with HIV-1. Magic Johnson volunteered to become a spokesperson for people with AIDS and this action was predicted to have great impact on young people as he endorsed the practice of safer sex. People of all ages became more aware of the risk of infection. The National AIDS Hotline increased from an average of 3800 calls a day to 40,000 the day Johnson made his announcement. The rate was even higher at the Centers for Disease Control, where there were 10,000 calls in one hour following the news broadcast. On November 7, 1991, when Johnson announced his retirement from basketball due to HIV-1 infection, one person with AIDS was dying every 15 minutes in the United States.

AIDS Research in the Early 1990s

Measuring disease progression became more accurate with continued research in the early 1990s. Studies demonstrated that the development of signs and symptoms of AIDS typically paralleled laboratory testing for CD4 lymphocytes (CDC, 1992a; Fahey et al, 1990). A decrease in the total CD4 count below 500/microliter was a precursor to the development of clinical AIDS. A drop below 200/microliter indicated the onset of clinical AIDS and a high probability for the development of AIDS-related opportunistic infections, neoplasms, or both. There appeared to be a low risk for death from HIV infection above the 200/microliter CD4 level. The CDC revised the classification system for HIV infection to emphasize the clinical importance of the CD4+ T-lymphocyte count in the categorization of HIV-related clinical conditions (CDC, 1992a).

Research studies revealed that one of HIV-1's major proteins, gag, unexpectedly binds to two human cellular proteins known as cyclophilins (Luban, Bossolt, Franke, Kalpana, & Goff, 1993). It already was known that certain drugs that bind cyclophilins, such as cyclosporin, an immunosuppressant used to prevent tissue rejection in organ transplantation, inhibited gag and cyclophilin binding. The possibility emerged that HIV-1 may exert its immune-suppressing activity by similarly binding to cyclophilins. These studies proposed that the knowledge of the gag-cyclophilin interaction should lead to the development of drugs that block the association, thus stopping HIV-1 proliferation and potentially preventing immune suppression. A difficulty with using this drug therapy is the added risk of giving an immunosuppressant to an individual with a compromised immune system.

Researchers at Columbia University used molecular biological tools that identified the region of the gag protein that allowed it to bind with cyclophilin (Luban et al., 1994). They altered the gag protein so one amino acid (proline) at position 222 was different. The mutated protein no longer bound cyclophilin and was not infectious. This finding led the way for development of a new class of drugs that inhibited binding of various cell surfaces to the HIV-1.

In December 1995, a research group led by Lusso and Gallo published findings about the identification of certain chemokines (proteins that help bring about inflammatory responses): RANTES, MIP-1α, and MIP-1β. The study results demonstrated that these chemokines are potent suppressers of HIV-1's ability to infect cells. This finding would play a pivotal role in future anti-HIV-1 drug development.

During the 1990s, there was rapid development of drug therapies that not only could prolong life but improve the quality of life for those individuals with HIV-1 and AIDS. As of December 1995, there were 28 FDA-approved drugs for HIV-1 infection and AIDS-related conditions (CDC, 1996b; NIH, 1990). In addition, there were 122 drugs being studied in HIV-1and AIDS clinical trials as of December 1995 (CDC, 1995e). Of those 122 drugs, 22 were potential vaccines.

Involvement of the CNS in HIV-1 and AIDS has been well documented for over a decade. HIV-1 crosses the blood-brain barrier and enters the nervous system early, probably concomitant with initial systemic infection (Resnick et al., 1985). The virus had been cultured from brain, nerve, and cerebrospinal fluid from persons at all stages of HIV disease, including those without neurologic signs or symptoms. Neuropathological studies had demonstrated that nearly all patients with AIDS have pathological abnormalities of the CNS. Involvement of the white matter and basal ganglia were first emphasized, such as was seen in HIV encephalitis or HIV leukoencephalitis. More recently, there was evidence that gray matter was involved (Ciardi et al., 1990; Levy & Berger, 1992). The cause of neuronal damage was unknown until the mid-1990s.

In 1995, Adle-Biassette and colleagues published findings about a mechanism that induced nerve cell death. Viral pathogenesis of the CNS had not been well understood up to this point. Scientists knew the virus did not directly infect the nerve cell because no HIV infection of neurons or glial cells had ever been found. Adle-Biassette and associates hypothesized that a lentivirus (especially HIV) may cause cell depletion and tissue atrophy in the brain, similar to its action on the immune system, by inducing **apoptosis** (a process in which a cell commits suicide). Autopsy results of 12 brains from adult individuals who had died at various stages of HIV-1 infection and four seropositive non-AIDS cases supported the hypothesis. The findings in the study showed that apoptosis was a constant finding in all 12 AIDS cases. In addition, it was noted that apoptotic neurons were present in generally equal amounts in the frontal lobe and temporal lobe.

Apoptosis is a physiological form of cell death that morphologically and biochemically differs from necrosis. It is a suicide mechanism that exists in healthy tissue and is essential for normal development, maturation, and turnover of tissues. Apoptosis is a process in which a cell commits suicide by disintegrating into particles that are then ingested by phagocyte cells. In individuals with intact immune systems, this process may be beneficial in limiting growth of tumor cells. Apoptosis is triggered by changes in the cellular environment and consequently the cell self-destructs. The presence of HIV in adjacent cells could precipitate the abnormal programmed cell death mechanism. The envelope glycoprotein gp120 is known to be neurotoxic and may be a contributing factor that triggers the cell suicide mechanism.

Current AIDS Research: 1996–1997

There were tremendous breakthroughs that occurred rapidly in 1996. In February, the journal *Science* published an article that summarized the key findings revealed at the 3rd Conference on Retroviruses and Opportunistic Infections held at the end of January 1996 (Cohen, 1996). The first two studies reported data on a new class of drugs called protease inhibitors. The third study reported on how viral load affected a person's survival.

The article discussed the study presented by Leonard, which focused on ritonavir, a protease inhibitor. Protease inhibitors are a class of drugs that block the activity of a protease enzyme needed for HIV-1 replication. Ritonavir had been tested in 1090 AIDS patients who had severely compromised immune systems. The CD4 counts in these individuals averaged 30 per cubic millimeter of blood whereas the normal counts range from 600 to 1200. Half of the cases received the drug and half received an inactive placebo during the 7-month study. Results showed that 33.1% of the placebo recipients developed an AIDS-related disease or died during the study period. In contrast, only 15.3% of the treated cases had similar outcomes. There were minimal side effects from the drugs, such as nausea and diarrhea. Further analysis indicated that ritonavir decreased the viral load sixfold through 16 weeks of trial, a relatively modest effect.

Another study discussed by Cohan (1996) presented findings on the protease inhibitor, indinavir. The research, done by Gulick and colleagues, placed 97 HIV-1 cases into three treatment groups: The control group received AZT plus 3TC (another reverse transcriptase inhibitor), the second group received indinavir alone, and the third group received all three drugs. The researchers found clinically significant differences in HIV-1 levels following the treatment. All study cases had more than 20,000 copies of HIV-1 RNA per milliliter of blood at the study's start. After 24 weeks, the viral RNA had plummeted 200-fold and was undetectable in 86% of the patients who received all three drugs. Only 40% of the cases receiving indinavir alone had undetectable virus levels. In the control group, using AZT and 3TC, HIV-1 was still easily detected in all cases. There were few reported serious side effects linked to indinavir use.

The findings of a third study also were discussed in the Cohan (1996) article. The researchers published their data in the same issue of *Science* (Mellors et al., 1996) as the Cohen summary. This study was conducted by Mellors and associates and investigated the use of viral load count (number of HIV-1 in the blood) to predict whether drug therapies help people live longer, healthier lives. The study concluded that the current standards of RNA counts or CD4 counts were adequate predictors. Mellors and associates analyzed blood samples collected every 6 months beginning as early as 1984 from each of 181 men, most of whom never took AZT or any other antiviral drug. After separating people by their initial viral loads and CD4 counts, the researchers assessed disease progression over several years. They found that the baseline viral load was the most accurate predictor of survival (Mellors et al., 1996).

Within a 6-week period in 1996, the discovery of two coreceptors of CD4 were announced. Researchers had known since 1986 that the presence of CD4 receptors alone was not sufficient for HIV-1 to gain entry into immune system cells (Maddon, 1986). This knowledge helped launch a decade-long search for a second coreceptor.

In May 1996, a research group led by Berger announced the discovery of a membrane protein they labeled fusin (Feng, Broder, Kennedy, & Berger, 1996). In experiments, the combination of fusin and CD4 allowed cells to fuse with HIV's surface, which is a key step in the infection process. HIV strains that infect T cells at later stages of the disease were shown to interact with fusin to gain entry into the immune cell. The discovery of fusin, in combination with the discovery of the chemokines (Cocci et al., 1995), opened possibilities for designing drugs that would block the fusin receptors directly or indirectly with the chemokines.

Within 6 weeks of the discovery of fusin came the discovery of another coreceptor: CC CKR 5 (Alkhatibet al., 1996; Deng et al., 1996; Dragic et al., 1996). These researchers identified CC CKR 5 as a cell membrane-bound protein that is a partner of HIV-1's primary receptor, CD4, in allowing HIV-1 to enter target cells in the critical early stages of infection.

The discovery of these coreceptors suggests that HIV-1 may use different molecules to enter the cell at different stages of the disease. The role of the coreceptors and chemokines also may explain why a small percentage of people, **exposed uninfected** (EU), have been able to resist HIV-1's ability to destroy the immune system even after being infected with HIV-1 for a decade. These individuals may have higher levels of chemokines, fewer fusin- or CC CKR 5-like receptors, or both.

The 11th International Conference on AIDS was held in Vancouver, Canada, in July 1996. Many of the findings of the previous months in 1996 were reiterated. However, for the first time, there was cautious optimism expressed by the participants of the conference about the future management of the HIV infection. The remainder of 1996 and early 1997 were characterized by studies that demonstrated the clinical benefits of improvements in antiretroviral therapy, especially in the management of opportunistic infections (CDC, 1997; Moore, Keruly, & Chaisson, 1997).

The research findings accomplished in 1996 marked a turning point in AIDS research and resulted in a paradigm shift—a new understanding of viral dynamics and the use of potent combination antiretroviral therapies to reduce and suppress HIV-1 in the blood. A new acronym began to be used in the scientific literature for this new drug therapy approach: HAART, or highly active antiretroviral therapy. HAART regimen demands strict compliance to the use of a combination of three to four protease inhibitor drugs for a sustained period of several years. It was hypothesized that if an individual responded to initial combined drug treatment by having HIV-1 levels in the blood drop to below measurable rates and CD4+ T-cell count rise significantly, then the HAART method would lead to eventual eradication of HIV-1 in the body in two to three years.

However, new data presented by Siliciano (1997) at the 37th Interscience Conference on Antimicrobial Agents and Chemotherapy (ICAAC) on September 28, 1997, brought disappointing news. Siliciano examined 22 individuals with HIV-1 infection who had been treated for as long as 30 months on 3–4 drug protease inhibitor-containing HAART regimens. All individuals demonstrated HIV-1 RNA suppression levels below 200 copies/mL. Testing was performed on resting lymphocytes, or latent cells. Of the 22 test subjects, four subjects had inadequate specimens for virus isolation. In the remaining 18, all were found to produce infectious virus upon stimulation by irradiation. The study further showed that the amount of time on HAART did not make a significant difference in the amount of infectious cells in the different test subjects. Since the latent HIV-1 cells could easily be stimulated to become active, the study results suggest that HIV-1 eradication may never be possible. However, an encouraging finding in this study was that no new mutations associated with drug resistance were found in the HIV-1 isolates. This suggests that suppression of replication with the combination regimens was sufficient to prevent the evolution of viral mutants. These data increase hope that long-term viral suppression is possible without the development of drug resistance. The researchers concluded that these data stress the importance of finding antiretroviral regimens that will be tolerable, effective, and affordable for long-term use.

At the end of 1997, no effective vaccine had yet been developed to protect against infection by HIV-1. At the 37th Interscience Conference on Antimicrobial Agents and Chemotherapy (ICAAC) in September, David Baltimore, Nobel laureate who had discovered the key retroviral enzyme reverse transcriptase and the new chairman of the NIH AIDS Vaccine Research Committee (AVRC), reviewed the current approaches to vaccine development. Baltimore (1997) outlined seven current approaches, stating that the best results to date have been achieved with a live attenuated vaccine using the simian immunodeficiency virus (SIV) in monkeys. However, Baltimore pointed out that, even though some of these animals resisted infection with a highly virulent strain of SIV subsequent to vaccination, the vaccine itself produced disease in some of the vaccinated monkeys.

The current funding by the United States government for vaccine development is in excess of $100 million a year (Baltimore, 1997). The National Institute of Allergy and Infectious Disease (NIAID) and National Cancer Institute are committed to constructing a joint vaccine laboratory at a vaccine-dedicated site by the year 2000.

AIDS DEMOGRAPHIC STUDIES

The AIDS epidemic continues to spread in the United States, but it has slowed significantly (CDC, 1995a; CDC, 1997). From 1981 through 1996, a total of 573,800 persons aged 13 years or older with AIDS were reported to the CDC by state and local health departments (CDC, 1997). From 1992 through 1996, non-Hispanic blacks, Hispanics, and women accounted for increasing proportions of persons reported with AIDS. In 1996, cases of AIDS reported in non-Hispanic blacks exceeded the proportion who were non-Hispanic white for the first time. The number of AIDS cases among women more than doubled, and reported cases of AIDS in heterosexuals more than tripled. As shown in Table 1–1, the demographics of AIDS is changing over time.

During the 1980s, HIV-1 infection emerged as one of the leading causes of death in the United States. Mortality data reported by the CDC for 1993 and 1994 indicates a continuing increase in HIV-1 infections as a leading cause of death in the United States, particularly among persons

Table 1–1. Demographic changes evident in AIDS adult target population.

Target Population	1981–1988	1993–Oct. 1995
Females	8%	18%
I. V. Drug Users	17%	27%
Homosexuals	64%	45%
Heterosexuals	3%	10%
Caucasians	60%	43%
African-Americans	25%	38%
Hispanics	14%	18%
Total Reported Cases During Time Period	**50,352**	**247,741**

Source: From data in "First 500,000 AIDS cases—United States, 1995" by the Centers of Disease Control and Prevention, 1995, *Morbidity and Mortality Weekly Report, 44,* p. 849.

aged 25–44 years (CDC, 1996a). Among persons in this age group, HIV-1 infection became the most common cause of death for African-American males in 1991.

By 1992, it was the leading cause of death for all men when combined as a category, and for Caucasian males in 1994. HIV-1 became the third leading cause of death among women in this age range in 1994. Table 1–2 summarizes the number and percentage of persons in the United States with AIDS, by selected demographic features, between 1981 to 1995.

For the first time in 1996, deaths among persons with AIDS decreased substantially. The decrease in deaths reflected better management of fatal opportunistic infections through improved medical care, increasing use of prophylactic drugs to prevent secondary infections, and the use of combination therapy with antiretroviral agents. In addition, the widespread availability of protease inhibitors, approved by the FDA in 1996, further improved the survival rate.

Despite these trends, during 1995, HIV-1 infection remained the leading cause of death among persons aged 25–44 years, accounting for 19% of deaths from all causes in this age group. The higher rate of opportunistic infections incidence rates among non-Hispanic blacks and Hispanics than among non-Hispanic whites may reflect reduced access to health care associated with disadvantaged socioeconomic status, cultural or language barriers that may limit access to prevention information, and differences in HIV risk behavior (CDC, 1997). The number of AIDS deaths did not decrease among women or persons infected through heterosexual contact. The incidence of cases associated with heterosexual contact has continued to increase, primarily reflecting transmission from the large population of intravenous drug users to their heterosexual partners.

CHAPTER SUMMARY

In June 1981, the Centers for Disease Control (CDC) reported the first cases of AIDS in the United States. This new illness was labeled a "gay disease" because the first victims were predominantly homosexual. During the early 1980s, the public believed that the proliferation of AIDS in the United States was due to gay males and their promiscuous sexual activities. This attitude impeded government support of research into AIDS and its treatment. By the late 1980s, the tide of public opinion had changed, and people were demanding more research about the disease and a possible cure. Since then, there has been a vast amount of research into HIV-1, but still there is no cure or vaccine.

From 1981 through 1996, nearly 600,000 persons have died from AIDS. The disease continues to spread in the United States but it has slowed significantly. In addition, there has been a change in the demo-

Table 1–2. Number and percentage of persons with AIDS, by selected characteristics and period of report.

Trait	1981–1987 No.	(%)	1988–1992 No.	(%)	1993–1995 No.	(%)	Cumulative No.	(%)
Sex								
Male	46,317	(92.0)	177,807	(87.5)	204,356	(82.5)	428,480	(85.5)
Female	4,035	(8.0)	25,410	(12.5)	43,383	(17.5)	72,828	(14.5)
Age Group								
0–4	653	(1.3)	2,766	(1.4)	2,013	(0.8)	5,432	(1.1)
5–12	100	(0.2)	669	(0.3)	616	(0.2)	1,385	(0.3)
13–19	199	(0.4)	758	(0.4)	1,343	(0.5)	2,300	(0.5)
20–29	10,531	(20.9)	38,662	(19.0)	41,861	(16.9)	91,054	(18.2)
30–39	23,269	(46.2)	92,493	(45.5)	111,992	(45.3)	227,754	(45.4)
40–49	10,491	(20.8)	7,088	(23.1)	64,990	(26.2)	122,569	(24.2)
50–59	3,690	(7.3)	14,537	(7.2)	18,413	(7.5)	36,640	(7.3)
≥e60	1,419	(2.8)	6,244	(3.1)	6,513	(2.6)	14,176	(2.8)
Race/Ethnicity								
White	30,104	(59.8)	102,551	(50.5)	105,516	(42.6)	238,171	(47.5)
Black	12,794	(25.44)	63,319	(31.2)	94,158	(38.0)	170,271	(34.0)
Hispanic	7,039	(14.0)	35,213	(17.3)	45,135	(18.2)	87,387	(17.4)
Asian	309	(0.6)	1,339	(0.7)	1,809	(0.7)	3,437	(0.7)
American Indian/ Alaskan Indian	67	(0.1)	433	(0.2)	783	(0.3)	1,283	(0.3)
HIV-Exposure Category								
Homosexual	32,246	(64.0)	110,934	(54.6)	111,257	(44.9)	254,437	(50.8)
IV drug user	8,639	(17.2)	49,093	(24.2)	67,708	(27.3)	125,440	(25.0)
Homosexual and IV drug user	4,193	(8.3)	14,252	(7.1)	13,984	(5.6)	32,429	(6.5)
Hemophiliac	505	(1.0)	1,744	(0.9)	2,009	(0.8)	4,258	(0.8)
Heterosexual	1,248	(2.5)	12,335	(6.1)	24,958	(10.1)	38,541	(7.7)
HIV-Exposure Category (continued)								
Transfusion recipients	1,285	(2.6)	3,894	(1.9)	2,521	(1.0)	7,700	(1.6)
Perinatal	608	(1.2)	3,084	(1.5)	2,432	(1.0)	6,124	(1.2)
No-risk reported	1,628	(3.2)	7,881	(3.9)	22,872	(9.2)	32,381	(6.4)
Region*								
Northeast	19,544	(38.3)	62,282	(30.6)	74,769	(30.2)	156,596	(31.2)
Midwest*	3,770	(7.5)	20,352	(10.0)	24,914	(10.1)	49,036	(9.8)
South*	12,960	(25.7)	65,926	(32.4)	86,462	(34.9)	165,348	(33.0)
West*	13,550	(26.9)	46,675	(23.0)	53,729	(21.7)	113,954	(22.7)
U.S. Territories	516	(1.0)	7,889	(3.9)	7,566	(3.1)	15,971	(3.2)

(continued)

Table 1–2. (*continued*).

Trait	1981–1987 No.	(%)	1988–1992 No.	(%)	1993–1995 No.	(%)	Cumulative No.	(%)
Vital Status								
Living	2,779	(5.5)	32,144	(15.8)	155,006	(62.6)	189,929	(37.9)
Deceased	47,573	(94.5)	171,073	(84.2)	92,735	(37.4)	311,381	(62.1)
Total	**50,352**	**(100.0)**	**203,217**	**(100.0)**	**247,741**	**(100.0)**	**501,310**	**(100.0)**

Note: **Northeast:** Connecticut, Maine, Massachusetts, New Hampshire, New Jersey, New York, Pennsylvania, Rhode Island, and Vermont. **Midwest:** Illinois, Indiana, Iowa, Kansas, Michigan, Minnesota, Missouri, Nebraska, North Dakota, Ohio, South Dakota, and Wisconsin. **South:** Alabama, Arkansas, Delaware, District of Columbia, Florida, Georgia, Kentucky, Louisiana, Maryland, Mississippi, North Carolina, Oklahoma, South Carolina, Tennessee, Texas, Virginia, and West Virginia. **West:** Alaska, Arizona, California, Colorado, Hawaii, Idaho, Montana, Nevada, New Mexico, Oregon, Utah, Washington, and Wyoming.
Source: From "First 500,000 AIDS Cases—United States, 1995" by Centers of Disease Control and Prevention, 1995, *Morbidity and Mortality Weekly Report, 44,* p. 850.

graphics of the target population. In the mid 1990s, women and minorities account for the largest percent increase in persons reported with AIDS, and reported cases in heterosexuals has more than tripled.

AIDS is an acronym for **acquired immunodeficiency syndrome**, a disease characterized by the slow destruction of the body's immune system. The agent that causes AIDS is **human immunodeficiency virus type 1**, or HIV-1. The terms AIDS and HIV-1 are not synonymous. AIDS refers to the end stages of an HIV-1 infection. The stages of HIV-1 disease are characterized by the presence of certain diseases.

2

Stages of HIV-1 Infection

There has been much research in medicine and biological sciences on the stages of HIV-1 infection. It is necessary for communication disorders professionals to understand the progression of the disease process and its identifiable stages. Therefore, a summary of information regarding disease progression and stages of disease in adults is presented in this chapter. This information covers expected clinical symptoms, as well as any known speech, language, or audiological involvement. The major stages of HIV-1 infection include transmission of HIV-1, acute, asymptomatic, early symptomatic, and late symptomatic. Although disease progression is similar in both adults and the pediatric population, there are some notable differences. These differences are discussed in Chapter 6.

Individuals exhibit great variance in the time spent in each stage. Based on extensive studies, researchers have determined the average duration of each stage. The usual course of HIV-1 infection is as follows:

- **Transmission of HIV-1:** Usually through sexual intercourse or blood exposure.
- **Acute Infection:** One to 6 weeks after transmission, during which an infectious mononucleosis-like illness develops. However, the person recovers in one to two weeks. Some people do not even notice this stage.
- **Seroconversion:** Four to 12 weeks, sometimes longer, during which the body develops antibodies to HIV-1. Consequently, the blood test for the presence of antibodies to HIV-1 is positive.
- **Asymptomatic Period:** This is a variable time interlude during which the person feels well and functions normally except for the

psychological stress accompanying the knowledge that he or she is HIV positive.

- **Early Symptomatic HIV-1 Infection:** Lasting 5 to 8 years, with considerable individual variation, in which the first symptoms or conditions that indicate weakening of the immune system, or **immunosuppression** appear. These conditions were previously termed AIDS-related complex (ARC).
- **Late Symptomatic HIV-1 Infection:** Eight to 10 years in which severe opportunistic infections and tumors occur. Research has shown that development of these opportunistic infections is such a reliable indicator of disease progression from HIV-1 infection to AIDS that they are now AIDS-defining diagnoses. Another criterion for an AIDS diagnosis is a CD4 cell count below 200.

TRANSMISSION OF HIV-1

HIV-1 is most frequently transmitted by all types of sexual contact, both heterosexual and homosexual. Other modes of infection include blood-to-blood contact or perinatal transmission from infected mothers to their infants. However, the predominant mode of HIV-1 transmission throughout the world is sexual contact.

HIV-1 has been identified in virtually every body fluid and tissue, including blood, semen, vaginal secretions, saliva, tears, breast milk, cerebrospinal fluid, amniotic fluid, urine, and fluid obtained from bronchoalveolar lavage (Saag, 1992). In most cases, the virus resides in **lymphocytes** (lymph cell or white blood corpuscle) that are present within the body fluids. Theoretically, any fluid that contains lymphocytes could be implicated in the spread of the virus. However, no cases of HIV-1 transmission have been reported through any body fluids except blood and blood products, fluids grossly contaminated with blood, semen, vaginal secretions, and, rarely, breast milk. HIV-1 has also been transmitted through transplanted organs, including kidney, liver, heart, pancreas, and bone.

When HIV-1 enters the body, it attaches itself only to CD4 receptors on the cell walls of CD4 cells. The **CD4** is a white blood cell, or a lymphocyte. (The CD4 cell is also called a *T4 cell* and a *T-helper cell.*) It belongs to a class of lymphocytes called **T cells,** which, along with **B cells,** are central parts of the immune system. The purpose of the CD4 cells is to coordinate the immune system's defense against a variety of infectious diseases.

Once HIV-1 attaches to a CD4 cell, it enters the cell and becomes part of the cell's genes. Genes are composed of DNA (deoxyribonucleic acid), a molecule that is responsible for directing the reproduction of the cell. A virus such as HIV-1 has only RNA (ribonucleic acid), a molecule that is actually a mirror image of DNA but that cannot produce new viruses. HIV-1 is a special virus called a **retrovirus,** meaning that it has a protein called reverse transcriptase. **Reverse transcriptase** allows the viral RNA to turn into a viral DNA that is capable of producing new HIV-1 instead of new CD4 cells. The virus eventually destroys the host CD4 cell, and the new viruses that have been produced then infect other CD4 cells. As the CD4 cells are infected and destroyed, the immune system functions less and less effectively, which is why the CD4 cell count is used as a criterion for measuring disease progression. HIV-1 is carried by CD4 cells and other lymphocytes to all parts of the body, including the brain. There also are certain cells in the brain that act as receptors for HIV-1.

ACUTE HIV-1 INFECTION

Acute infection of HIV-1 is sometimes referred to as a mononucleosis-like syndrome because many of the symptoms of acute infection resemble those of infectious mononucleosis. However, a blood test for mononucleosis will be negative because the symptoms are caused by a different virus.

The first symptoms of HIV-1 infection occur early in the disease process. The interval between transmission of the virus and the first symptoms of acute infection lasts, on average, between one and six weeks. The symptoms of early HIV-1 infection include fever, sweats, malaise, fatigue, achiness, joint pain, headaches, dysphagia or odynophagia (pain during swallowing), and enlarged lymph glands (Bartlett & Finkbeiner, 1993). Some individuals may exhibit a rash over the chest, back, and abdomen. Rarely, some individuals may experience temporary upper or lower limb paresis or paralysis.

Individuals may demonstrate evidence of infection of the brain, including severe headaches, mood changes, personality changes, irritability, and confusion. Early neurologic complications may evolve acutely or subacutely and may take the form of focal or diffuse encephalitis or leukoencephalopathy. Meningitis, ataxia, or myelopathy, either alone or concomitant with peripheral nervous system abnormalities, may be present (Price, Brew, & Roke, 1992; Worley & Price, 1992). Most individuals recover from these disorders within a number of weeks. However, in some patients with encephalitis, residual cognitive deficits may exist (Worley & Price, 1992).

The duration of acute HIV-1 infection usually lasts one or two weeks. There are some individuals who have no symptoms of an acute infection stage. Many people infected with HIV-1 mistake the early symptoms for a common viral infection. A minority of people feel sick enough to go to a physician. Occasionally, people experience excessive fatigue that lasts weeks or months.

A physician will find enlarged lymph glands and an enlarged spleen. Results of blood tests will reveal fewer white blood cells than normal. Liver tests may indicate changes suggesting mild hepatitis. A spinal tap to analyze cerebrospinal fluid may show evidence of meningitis. However, many conditions can be responsible for these test results. If a blood test to detect antibodies to HIV-1 is done during early acute HIV-1 infection stage, the results will be negative. That is because it usually takes four to twelve weeks after transmission for the antibodies to appear in the blood in sufficient concentration to result in a positive test (Walker, 1992).

During the acute infection stage, if a blood test for measuring the presence of HIV-1 (not the antibody) is done, it would be positive. The viremia (viral load) of HIV-1 is very high during this stage because the body has no mechanism to fight it. Soon after infection, the level of viremia rapidly decreases when the antibodies to HIV-1 develop.

SEROCONVERSION

The body takes several days to weeks to recognize a foreign substance like a virus. Once the immune system is alerted, certain white blood cells, called *B lymphocytes,* produce serum proteins, or **antibodies,** to attack the foreign matter. The appearance of antibody response is called **seroconversion.** Seroconversion generally occurs four to twelve weeks after transmission, but in rare cases it may take up to a year (Bartlett & Finkbeiner, 1993; Walker, 1992). For unknown reasons, the virus appears to be dormant in these individuals so the immune system is not manufacturing antibodies against it.

Antibodies against most viruses eliminate the virus and then stay in the body to protect against future infections by the same virus. Virtually all people with HIV-1 infection develop antibodies against HIV-1. These antibodies reduce concentration of the HIV-1 but do not eliminate HIV-1. As a result, persons with HIV-1 remain infected and capable of transmitting the virus for life.

ASYMPTOMATIC HIV-1 INFECTION OF THE CNS

For several years after seroconversion, people with HIV-1 infection may remain asymptomatic. During this period, the person will be unaware of the HIV-1 infection unless a blood test shows antibodies to the virus. It is estimated that 70–80% of the people who presently are infected are in this asymptomatic phase (Bartlett & Finkbeiner, 1993). The duration of this stage is highly variable. The average is 5 to 8 years until the symptoms of HIV-1 infection appear, and 8 to 10 years until AIDS is diagnosed.

HIV-infected individuals are regarded as asymptomatic only if there is no history of HIV-related opportunistic infections or malignancies and no symptoms compatible with AIDS-related complex (ARC). Since there is a period of several years after initial infection during which the individual remains asymptomatic, it was once believed that a latent phase of HIV-1 infection existed.

Recent studies have shown that there is no true latent period in the disease process (Gray et al., 1993; Neunen-Jacob et al., 1996). Neuronal cell death and demyelinating neuropathies have been noted in fully functional, asymptomatic individuals who have remained well for a year or more. These neuropathies resemble Guillain-Barré syndrome or chronic inflammatory demyelinating polyneuropathy (CIDP) except that the HIV-1-related demyelinization has an autoimmune basis.

HIV-1 has been shown to penetrate the blood-brain barrier early in the course of infection and can be found in the cerebrospinal fluid (CSF) in almost half of infected individuals before the development of any of the medical symptoms of HIV-defining illnesses (Stern, Silva, Chaisson, & Evans, 1996). Autopsy studies also have revealed that significant neuronal cell death occurs in the basal ganglia in the asymptomatic phase of HIV infection (Neunen-Jacob et al., 1996). Growing evidence now suggests that subclinical or mild neuropsychological impairments can be detected in 25–34% of asymptomatic individuals (Heaton et al., 1994; Stern et al., 1996; Stout et al., 1995). However, a few studies have found a low prevalence of neuropsychological deficits in the early stages of HIV-1 infection (McArthur et al., 1989; Miller et al., 1990).

Nutritional alterations are widespread during the early asymptomatic stages of HIV-1 infection. The nutritional imbalances are due to factors such as malabsorption of nutrients due to cell changes occurring in the body. Many neurological symptoms, ranging from peripheral neuropathies to global cognitive impairment, have been demonstrated as a consequence of nutritional and metabolic imbalance in HIV-1 infection (Chelbowski, Grosvenor, Bernhard, Morales, & Bulcavage, 1989). A 4-year longitudinal study of 84 HIV-1-infected homosexual men in the asymptomatic phase has demonstrated significant negative effect on information processing speed that occurred due to the imbalance of a single chemical, cobalamin, in the brain (Shor-Posner, Morgan, Whilkie, Eisdorfer, & Baum, 1995). Frequently, multiple chemicals are imbalanced in an individual with HIV-1 infection (Beach et al., 1992).

Follow-up care during the asymptomatic phase is crucial. Due to the multisystemic nature of HIV-1 infection and the numerous associated clinical disorders described in Table 2–1, it is imperative that a consistent program of screening, testing, immunological staging, therapy, and subspecialty consultation be implemented. A thorough neurological assessment directed toward detecting evidence of peripheral neuropathy (motor

Table 2–1. Common nonspecific signs and symptoms of HIV-1 infection.

General	***Gastrointestinal (continued)***
Fever	Odynophagia
Weight loss	Jaundice
Generalized lymphadenopathy	Spleen infection
Dermatological	Liver infection
Ulcerations	***Musculoskeletal***
Pustules	Arthritis
Nodules	Arthralgias
Ocular	Reiter's syndrome
Decreased visual acuity	***Neurological***
Visual field deficit	Headache
Periocular skin lesions	Seizures
Retinal hemorrhage, exudates	***Cognitive Dysfunction***
Dry eyes	Inattention
Oral	Reduced concentration
Candidiasis/ulcerations	Forgetfulness
Nodules/sarcomas	***Motor Dysfunction***
Thrush	Slowed movements
Parotid gland enlargement	Clumsiness
Periodontal disease	Ataxia
Dry mouth	***Behavioral Manifestation***
Hairy leukoplakia	Apathy
Gastrointestinal	Altered personality
Diarrhea	Depression
Dysphagia	

Source: From "Associated communications disorders and dysphagia in adults with HIV-1 and secondary CNS lesions" by C. R. Larsen, 1996, p. 47. Unpublished master's independent study, University of North Dakota, Grand Forks.

and sensory examination, deep tendon flexes), focal neurological deficits (cognitive decline, decreased short-term memory, difficulty concentrating), and myelopathy should be done every 3 to 6 months.

EARLY SYMPTOMATIC HIV-1 INFECTION

Early symptomatic HIV-1 infection is the stage in which the first symptoms of a weakened immune system occur. Sometimes this stage of infection is referred to as AIDS-related complex, or ARC. The conditions usually are less severe than those used to define AIDS but not in all individuals. The onset may or may not indicate the immune system is weakening.

Several systems of classification are used to track the course of infection. The system used by the United States government is the CD4 cell count classification system. The Centers for Disease Control has updated this system several times since 1982 to add to the criterion more diseases recognized as being associated with HIV-1 infection. The revised classification system for HIV infection is based on the recommended clinical standard of monitoring CD4+ T-lymphocyte counts, because this parameter consistently correlates with HIV-related immune dysfunction and disease progression. However, HIV-1-infected adolescents and adults are categorized on the basis of clinical conditions associated with HIV infection and CD4+ T-lymphocyte counts.

Normal CD4 cell count is approximately 1000 CD4 cells in each cubic milliliter of blood. During the asymptomatic stage, the number of CD4 cells in infected individuals decreases every year as the virus continues its destruction. When the first symptoms occur in the early symptomatic HIV-1 infection stage, the CD4 cell count is between 200 to 499. For many people, the CD4 cell count is less than 300 when symptoms occur in this stage. When the cell count becomes low enough, the immune system is so compromised that it cannot fight off viral, bacterial, and parasitic attacks.

The most common conditions in this stage are thrush, oral hairy leukoplakia, shingles, idiopathic thrombocytopenic purpura, pneumonia, gynecological problems, and constitutional symptoms, which include fatigue, chronic fever, weight loss, and chronic diarrhea (CDC, 1992a; Dichtel, 1992; Phelan, 1997). All of these conditions are experienced by people who are not infected with HIV-1, but in the infected individuals, the conditions are chronic because they persist for several weeks or months.

The oral manifestations common to this stage of infection negatively affect mastication and swallow. In addition, the chronic constitutional conditions contribute to metabolic imbalances that affect cognition. Medications used to combat opportunistic infections frequently are ototoxic, causing sensorineural hearing loss. These issues will be addressed in more detail in the following chapters.

LATE SYMPTOMATIC HIV-1 INFECTION OR AIDS

The late symptomatic stage is one of severe immunosuppression. The CD4 cell count is less than 200 and the individual is vulnerable to serious opportunistic infections and tumors. Also, in the late stages of HIV-1 infection when immune defenses have been severely compromised and systemic complications have begun to accumulate, the nervous system becomes highly susceptible to a wide array of disorders involving the meninges, brain, spinal cord, peripheral nerves, and muscles.

Recent neuroimaging and neuropathology studies have demonstrated that the white matter, deep gray matter (basal ganglia and thalamus), and mesial temporal lobe structures are especially vulnerable to the effects of HIV-1 infection (Neuen-Jacob et al., 1996). These data indicate that HIV-1 most frequently damages the subcortical regions of the brain that are associated with attention, learning, and memory functions.

Despite early infection of the CNS, notable symptoms of cognitive impairment typically occur late in symptomatic HIV-1 disease. The most debilitating of the neurological disorders in late disease stage is HIV-1-associated dementia complex (ADC). ADC primarily affects the subcortical structures of the brain (basal ganglia, thalamus, cerebellum, and brain stem) and manifests itself as a progressive dementia that may be accompanied by cognitive, motor, and behavioral dysfunction (Price et al., 1988; Price, Brew, & Roke, 1992). The dementia is characterized by mental and verbal slowness, inattention, loss of concentration, and short-term memory loss (Maruff et al., 1994).

Apart from dementia, HIV-1-infected individuals are at risk for a wide range of neurologic diseases. Diffuse or global cerebral disease can result in altered mental status or generalized seizures. Focal disease often produces hemiparesis, hemisensory loss, visual field cuts, or disturbances in language use. Fungal, viral, and mycobacterial meningoencephalitis, lymphoma, and progressive multifocal leukoencephalopathy account for the majority of focal presentations. The spinal cord is affected by viral and, less frequently, fungal and parasitic opportunistic infections. Systemic lymphoma can infiltrate nerve roots and meninges.

In adults infected with HIV-1, impairment of voluntary motor activity can occur as a sign of extrapyramidal involvement preceding overt clinical signs and symptoms of motor system dysfunction (Arendt, Maecker, Purrman, & Homberg, 1994). Speech and swallowing disorders have been noted in these CNS pathologies.

Progressive deficits in cognition affect language ability in the symptomatic phase by reducing information processing speed (Shor-Posner et al., 1995), executive function, working memory, and attention (Kieburtz et al., 1996; Maruff et al., 1994). Language is primarily a cortical function and appears to remain mostly intact in individuals with HIV-1 infection until the very end stage of the disease process when global cognitive deficits are manifested. This is consistent with findings that show HIV-1 primarily affects subcortical regions of the brain (Masliah et al., 1992; Petito, Cho, Lemann, Navia, & Price, 1986; Vinters & Anders, 1990).

The dominant medical problems of the late stage of HIV-1 infection are opportunistic infections and tumors. Most opportunistic infections are caused by microbes to which everyone is exposed on a regular basis. However, these infections are frequently fatal due to the severe immunosuppression at this stage. *Pneumocystis carinii pneumonia* and Kaposi's sarcoma are the most common of the opportunistic infections. Less frequently occurring infections are tuberculosis, *Mycobacterium avium intracellulare,* *Toxoplasma gondii,* cryptococcosis, cytomegalovirus, herpes simplex, and cryptosporidiosis. These conditions, and others that affect speech, language, cognition, hearing, or swallow function, will be discussed in Chapters 4, 5, and 6.

CHAPTER SUMMARY

People who are infected with HIV-1 experience a slow deterioration of their immune system. The immune system is critical to proper functioning of the human body. When the immune system becomes compromised, the body is at risk for infection and disease. The human immune system has many different components that work together cooperatively to protect the body. HIV-1 attacks one particular part of the immune system, a type of white blood cell called CD4 cells (also called T helper, T4, or T cells). People with HIV-1 infection are particularly at risk for certain specific types of infections and cancers (opportunistic infections). In a person with an intact immune system, the fungal, bacterial, and parasitic agents that cause opportunistic infections ordinarily are controlled by CD4 cell function. Once sufficient numbers of CD4 cells are destroyed, the body loses its defense system against these common pathogens.

HIV-1 can also infect brain cells, cells inside bone marrow, and cells that line the digestive tract. Infection of brain cells causes changes in mental status by altering memory, cognition, and personality. As a result of HIV-1 infection of bone marrow, cells that produce blood die, leading to decreased blood counts and anemia. Symptoms of anemia include lethargy, weakness, headache, oral lesions, and gastrointestinal disturbances. HIV-1 infection of the lining of the gastrointestinal tract leads to dysphagia, odynophagia, chronic diarrhea, weight loss, and gastrointestinal disturbances.

The average time from infection with HIV-1 to developing full-blown AIDS is between eight to ten years. Individuals exhibit great variance in the time spent in each stage. The usual course of HIV-1 infection is as follows:

- **Transmission of HIV-1:** usually through sexual intercourse or blood exposure.
- **Acute Infection:** One to six weeks after transmission during which an infectious mononucleosis-like illness develops.
- **Seroconversion:** Four to twelve weeks, sometimes longer, during which the body develops antibodies to HIV-1.

- **Asymptomatic Period:** This is a variable time interlude during which the person feels well and functions normally except for the psychological stress accompanying the knowledge that he or she is HIV positive.
- **Early Symptomatic HIV-1 Infection:** Lasting five to eight years, with considerable individual variation, in which the first symptoms or conditions that indicate weakening of the immune system, or *immunosuppression* appear. These conditions were previously termed AIDS-related complex (ARC).
- **Late Symptomatic HIV-1 Infection:** Eight to ten years in which severe opportunistic infections and tumors occur. A criterion for an AIDS diagnosis is a CD4 cell count below 200.

 **3**

Clinical Management of Clients with HIV-1 Infection

It is imperative that speech-language pathologists (SLPs) and audiologists become more knowledgeable about HIV-1 infection. Surveys of hospitals in 1992 revealed that the incidence of HIV-infection in the patient population varied from 0.1 to 7.8%. Between 1993 to 1995, there were over 4000 cases of HIV/AIDS reported in children from ages 0 to 18 years in the United States, and the incidence in this age group is growing. This suggests that whether SLPs and audiologists work in the medical setting or the school setting, they will become more involved in the management issues surrounding the disease. The dilemmas created by AIDS that have challenged other health care workers soon will be confronting a larger number of the professionals in communication disorders.

The multisystemic nature of the disease has precipitated the trend toward multi- and interdisciplinary team approach to management of individuals with HIV-1 infection. SLPs and audiologists must become informed about all aspects of HIV-infection that affect their effectiveness as clinicians. In addition, the task of educating the public about the ramifications of early CNS involvement in disease progression and its impact on speech, language, cognition, hearing, and swallowing should be undertaken by SLPs and audiologists.

CHANGING ROLE OF SLPS AND AUDIOLOGISTS

In the past, referral for speech-language pathology and audiology services did not occur until the end stages of AIDS. Prior to the recent success of new drugs, patients died rapidly during the end stages of the disease. Patients were often chronically and acutely ill; therefore, therapy for speech, language, cognition, and hearing impairments was not a priority. Primary care providers were concerned mainly with the life-threatening illnesses that plagued their patients. Dysphagia complaints commonly were addressed by gastroenterologists.

As the latest statistics from the Centers for Disease Control (1997) substantiate, prophylactic interventions are now reducing the incidence of the often lethal opportunistic infections, increasing the average life expectancy. As people with HIV-1 live longer, there is greater likelihood that disorders of communication will have greater relevance to that population. Longer life spans will mean that individuals with HIV-1 infection will become more concerned with maintaining a productive and meaningful life for as long as possible. People need these skills to remain employed, maintain a productive lifestyle, and to make or keep social and personal contacts.

The communication and swallowing impairments associated with HIV-1 infection frequently are neurogenic in nature. Research has shown that even while individuals are asymptomatic and there are no overt signs of disease progression, there is subtle damage occurring to the CNS. Dysarthria, apraxia, progressive dementia, and sensorineural hearing loss are some of the impairments found in this client population. Subtle cognitive changes or reductions in short-term memory functioning and executive functioning have been noted. Others may experience some impairment of fine motor control necessary for speech or writing. Still others may experience impaired communicative effectiveness due to deficits in motor and sensory integration.

In addition to deficits in cognition, speech, hearing, language skills, and swallow function also are affected by HIV-1 infection. The early CNS involvement and changing pattern of opportunistic infections have been shown to compromise the auditory nerve (Ollo, Johnson, & Graftman, 1991). There is growing evidence of both central and peripheral hearing loss associated with opportunistic infections such as Kaposi's sarcoma (Dichtel, 1992; Flower & Sooy, 1987; Lalwani & Sooy, 1992). Dysphagia and odynophagia are common complaints of many individuals and have been shown to occur at all stages of infection. In one study of 71 adult males with HIV-1 infection, dysphagia was noted in 21% of the cases (Chelbowski et al., 1989).

NEED FOR MULTIDISCIPLINARY TEAM APPROACH

General care of individuals infected with HIV-1 has undergone a transformation since the first cases of infection were reported in 1981. HIV-1 infection was perceived as a rare disorder for which care was provided largely by physicians specializing in infectious diseases, clinical immunology, oncology, and dermatology. Since the full spectrum of pathologies associated with HIV-1 has become known, it has become clear that the relatively small numbers of primary care and allied health care clinicians specializing in AIDS would be unable to provide care for the hundreds of thousands of persons infected with the virus.

The numerous diverse manifestations of HIV-1 infection have led to increasing involvement of other specialties and subspecialties. Examples of these include ophthalmology, neurology, psychiatry, nephrology, gastroenterology, hematology, rheumatology, otorhinolaryngology, audiology, and speech-language pathology. There is a growing need for specialists who not only are knowledgeable about HIV infection, but are willing and able to effectively coordinate multidisciplinary approaches to therapy. Ready access to specialty and subspecialty consultants may greatly facilitate the care of HIV-infected individuals at all stages of the disease.

CASE MANAGEMENT

Speech-language pathologists (SLPs) and audiologists still are not typically involved in the management of individuals with HIV-1 infection early in the course of the disease process. A growing body of evidence has demonstrated that mild impairments of speech, language, hearing, or swallowing function may present at any stage of the disease (Belman, 1992; Diamond & Cohen, 1992; Flower & Sooy, 1987; Friedman, 1994; Jenkins, 1996; Kwartler et al., 1991; Lalwani & Sooy, 1992; Pressman, 1992; Straus, 1997). For this reason, communication disorders specialists should participate in the initial evaluation of the individual with HIV-1 infection. Education of other health care professionals and the public is necessary to increase the diagnostic role played by SLPs and audiologists.

For most individuals infected with HIV-1, communicative competence and swallowing function remain mostly intact until the more advanced stages of HIV infection. The end-stage frequently is characterized by progressive dementia, depression, immobilization, and malnutrition requiring intubation. Referrals for services from our profession are more common at this phase. SLPs who provide dysphagia therapy may become involved earlier than those clinicians who work primarily with the cognitive or motor deficit components of the infection.

The ability to maintain effective communication as long as possible is crucial to individuals with progressive debilitating disease. Better public awareness of the early signs of speech, language, hearing, and swallowing impairments that are associated with HIV-1 should increase the number of consultations and referrals made for speech, language, cognition, hearing, and dysphagia services at earlier stages of disease progression.

Service delivery settings for adults with HIV-1 infection will depend on their current health status. Emergency hospitalization frequently is necessary in the advanced stages. However, as the number of HIV-infected persons requiring hospitalization has grown, increasing emphasis has been placed on providing some services in the home if the individual can be hospitalized on short notice. Hospitalization in an acute care facility may be inappropriate for those who do not need diagnostic or intensive nursing care. If available, long-term care facilities or hospices may be more appropriate in those cases.

In the absence of research to indicate otherwise, it is assumed that treatment procedures currently used in the cases of motor speech disorders, language impairments, cognitive deficits, dementia, hearing impairments, and swallowing difficulties may be applied to patients with HIV-1 infection. The etiology of the communication disorders is HIV-1 infection; however, the bases for the impairments are the secondary CNS involvement and/or structural manifestations. Currently, due to the lack of published research or efficacy data, it would be pretentious to promote a specific case management plan for patients with HIV-1 infection. Therefore, there is a need for treatment efficacy research involving patients with HIV-1 infection.

BASES OF AIDS-RELATED
COMMUNICATION DISORDERS

Flower and Sooy (1987) published the first data about AIDS-related communication disorders. They discussed the bases of communication disorders frequently seen in individuals with AIDS (Table 3–1). Data gathered from 399 cases at the University of California-San Francisco revealed that one in eight cases showed lesions in the mouth, pharynx, and larynx due to Kaposi's sarcoma. In these cases, dysphonia could occur, but articulation was not affected. More frequently, the communication disorders were attributable to neurological components associated with AIDS. These included motor speech disorders as well as language disorders. Other symptoms evident in these cases were apathy, forgetfulness, withdrawal, cognitive deterioration, and depression. Flower and Sooy noted that, during the late stages of AIDS, the use of respirators and intubation further complicated the communication process for these individuals.

In 1991, Flower authored a chapter in a book titled *Rehabilitation for Patients with HIV Disease* that discussed multidisciplinary rehabilitative services for individuals with HIV and AIDS. Flower reported that individ-

Table 3–1. Manifestations of AIDS that underlie communication disorders.

Neurologic Manifestations

- opportunistic infections that attack CNS,
- AIDS-related dementia,
- peripheral and cranial neuropathies,
- tumors that impact the neurologic function of individuals, and
- cognitive and personality changes due to depression and CNS pathology.

Ear, Nose, and Throat Manifestations

- middle ear pathologies,
- ABR abnormalities,
- conductive and sensorineural hearing loss,
- vocal quality pathology,
- viral and fungal infections found in the ear, nose, throat, and mouth,
- lymphomas and tumors that impact hearing and speech, and
- hypopharyngeal and laryngeal function problems due to tumors and infection.

---

uals with AIDS were living longer. She predicted that speech-language pathologists would become involved in case management earlier than in the past. Historically, speech-language pathologists had become involved at the late stages of the disease when an individual needed an augmentative system to communicate due to loss of cognitive functions, motor functions, or both.

The major neuropathologic manifestations of HIV-1 can be broadly divided into three classifications according to neuroanatomic localization: (1) brain, (2) meninges, and (3) spinal cord. Where applicable, this classification can be further subdivided into whether the lesions are predominantly nonfocal or focal, and uncommon or common.

Among the manifestations of HIV-1 infection are an array of clinically important and diverse disorders. Communication disorders and dysphagia arise from secondary lesions to the CNS, opportunistic infections, and structural obstruction caused by lymphomas. The psychological affect of infection and disease progression are profound.

The primary CNS disorder associated with HIV-1 is AIDS dementia, which is variously termed AIDS dementia complex (ADC), HIV cognitive-motor complex, and HIV encephalopathy (HIVE). Other effects of HIV-1 on the CNS include profound immunosuppression and consequent opportunistic infections, autoimmunity, secondary consequences of systemic organ dysfunction (e. g., hypoxic encephalopathy), and drug toxicities of therapies associated with the HIV-1 infection. These will be discussed in greater detail in Chapter 4.

The latest data released by the Centers for Disease Control (CDC, 1997) reveal that for the first time, deaths among persons with AIDS have decreased substantially. The decrease in AIDS deaths reflects both the successful medical management of HIV-related opportunistic infections and improved survival among persons with AIDS. Increasing survival reflects recent improvements in medical care, the use of combination therapy with antiretroviral agents, and increasing use of prophylactic drugs to prevent secondary opportunistic infections. In addition, the widespread availability of protease inhibitors, approved by the Food and Drug Administration in 1996, may improve survival further. This increased survival rate indicates the growing need for medical and other allied services for persons with HIV-1 infection.

OCCUPATIONAL EXPOSURE TO HIV-1

A topic that is relevant in a discussion about the clinical management of clients with HIV-1 infection is the concern over occupational exposure. Fear of being exposed to a fatal disease is a legitimate concern. Although the risk of HIV-1 transmission to speech-language pathologists and audiologists is relatively small, there is still concern about occupational exposure.

Occupational exposures include contact of the eyes, mouth, other mucous membranes, broken skin, and subcutaneous contact with infected blood or other infectious materials (CDC, 1987; CDC, 1992b; CDC, 1995d). All clinicians should be knowledgeable about the natural history of HIV-1 infection and its clinical signs and symptoms. Increased awareness of risks to exposure in the clinical setting will minimize the danger of exposure. Well informed clinicians will more readily establish strategies to diminish the incidence of skin and mucous membrane exposure to bodily fluids and secretions, thereby reducing their risk of exposure to the virus.

Risk of Transmission to Health Care Workers

In late 1984, while using a gas syringe, a nurse in Great Britain became infected with HIV-1 as a consequence of accidental injection of fresh blood from a person with AIDS (Anonymous, 1984). Since then, documentation of HIV-1 transmission to health care and laboratory workers have been published by multiple investigators around the world (Weiss, 1997). Transmission to health care workers has occurred from several types of HIV-1 exposure: contaminated hollow bore and solid needles, other cuts, mucosal splashes, and skin contact with contaminated blood or body fluids.

There is currently much epidemiologic evidence that HIV-1 transmission has been demonstrated in association with blood, semen, cervicovaginal secretions, and breast milk (Weiss, 1997). However, HIV-1 has been detected in many other body fluids. These include cerebrospinal fluid, pleural fluid, sputum, nasal secretions, cerumen, tears, sweat, vomitus, and saliva (Groopman et al., 1984). There has been no evidence of HIV-1 transmission from these fluids alone although controversy exists about the role of saliva (Vidmar et al., 1996; Weiss, 1997). In the dental setting, saliva invariably is contaminated with blood and is treated as infectious. Currently, the Centers for Disease Control and Prevention does not include saliva alone among the list of body fluids for which universal precautions should apply (CDC, 1987; CDC, 1992b; CDC, 1995d).

The vast majority of occupational exposures to HIV-1 occurred **percutaneously,** or effected through the skin. This may occur when the live virus comes in contact with broken skin, by injection of a tainted needle through the skin, or a cut by an instrument that had come into contact with HIV-1 infected body fluid. **Mucocutaneous** occupational exposure, or mucous membrane to skin contact, has been reported, but rarely.

As of June 1996, 51 documented and 108 possible cases of occupationally acquired HIV-1 infection had been reported in the United States to the Centers for Disease Control (CDC, 1996d). According to an analysis of data pooled from 21 prospective studies, the risk associated with occupational exposure to HIV-1 through percutaneous exposure to blood from an infected patient, such as a needle stick or cut from a scalpel, or other contaminated devices was 0.2% (9 cases of HIV-1 infection that resulted from 3628 exposures) (Gerberding, 1995).

The most at-risk group of health care workers are those that deal directly with blood, blood products, or body fluids contaminated by blood. However, the task of calculating risk among individual workers is difficult because the variables influencing transmissibility have not been clearly identified. Factors that are theorized to affect risk from percutaneous or mucocutaneous exposure are summarized in Table 3–2.

In late 1995, the CDC reported a summary of an analysis of selected health care workers who showed seroconversion due to occupational exposure to HIV-1 (CDC, 1995d). The results showed an increased risk of HIV-1 transmission from exposure events in which high viral load exposure was likely. The highest viral load is found in blood and blood products of infected individuals during the acute infection stage, before seroconversion, and at the last stages of AIDS. Because neither the person in the acute infection stage nor the health care worker knows the person is infected with HIV-1, it is imperative that clinicians treat all clients with equal precaution.

In addition to exposure to HIV-1 through blood and body fluids, health care workers face exposure to secondary infections related to

Table 3–2. Factors influencing risk of acquiring HIV-1 infection from percutaneous or mucocutaneous occupational exposure.

Percutaneous Exposure	*Mucocutaneous Exposure*
Viral load in contaminant	Viral load in contaminant
Source/patient's disease stage	Volume of contaminant
Volume of contaminant involved	Duration of contact/exposure
Type/gauge of needle in exposure	Portal of entry of contaminant
Depth of penetration of needle	Intactness of skin of exposed worker
Whether latex gloves were worn	State of exposed worker's immune
State of exposed worker's immune	system
system	

HIV-1. There is increasing evidence that opportunistic infections may be spread in urban settings and in hospitals via air-borne pathogens (Sepkowitz, 1996). The possibility of **no ocomial** (pertaining to a hospital or infirmary) outbreaks of several infectious agents have been described, including *Pneumocystis carinii* (Jacobs et al., 1991; Walzer, 1991); *Mycobacterium tuberculosis* (DiPerri et al., 1989); and pneumococcal infections (Weiss, 1997).

Many forms of secondary infections develop into drug-resistant strains. There is a documented case of a health care worker whose death was attributed to occupational acquisition of multiply drug-resistant tuberculosis (CDC, 1991). As the AIDS epidemic progresses, it is likely that new resistance patterns will emerge, posing a health threat to health care providers in the future.

The issue of air-borne pathogens has important ramifications in a hospital setting due to the design and adequacy of ventilating systems in these institutions. Adherence to infection control guidelines will be imperative to minimize these problems.

Risks to Speech-Language Pathologists and Audiologists

Speech-language pathologists (SLPs) and audiologists are not at an increased risk for exposure to HIV-1. The virus has been isolated infrequently in the following body fluids and secretions that clinicians may come into contact with: cerumen, nasal secretions, saliva, sweat, and tears. Current research generally indicates that these pose minimal risks, as transmission of HIV-1 through these fluids does not occur routinely. However, as noted in the above section, there is controversy regarding the role of saliva in HIV-1 transmission.

There is now documented evidence of HIV-1 transmission through saliva alone in several cases (Murray et al., 1991; Vidmar et al., 1996). In two of these studies, HIV-1 occurred as a result of a bite. There is also evidence that persons with HIV-1 infection are prone to periodontal disease and oral lesions that increase the likelihood of blood in the saliva. It is generally accepted that saliva contaminated with blood should be treated as blood itself (Weiss, 1997). In light of this data, this author recommends that saliva should be treated in the same manner as blood itself until further evidence to the contrary can be provided.

Precautions in the Clinic Setting

Prevention of HIV-1 transmission can be achieved through appropriate attention to personal barrier measures, proper handling and cleaning of instruments, and sanitary disposal of contaminated waste materials. Intact skin blocks the virus, but small cuts and abrasions that may go unnoticed may pose risks. If the clinician is unsure of the skin's condition, rinsing of the hands with alcohol will reveal abrasions (because these will sting). The use of gloves provides an adequate personal barrier.

Unsterile examination gloves are required for all examinations and procedures that contact mucous membranes or secretions. After use, these must then be disposed of appropriately. General purpose utility gloves are adequate for clean-up of environmental surfaces and instruments. The utility gloves may be used again if they are adequately cleansed after use. Handwashing between patient contacts is mandatory. Due to frequent handwashing, the skin may become dry and chapped; therefore, using hand lotion may be beneficial.

The use of goggles is recommended if in close proximity to a patient during head and neck examination. Protective glasses, goggles, or face shields are warranted when there is a possibility of patients coughing up secretions, such as in intubations and tracheostomies. Laryngoscopy and endoscopic procedures under local anesthesia are associated with midfacial splatter by secretions, particularly to the eye of the examiner.

The Centers for Disease Control and Prevention (CDC, 1987) has published recommendations for prevention of HIV in health care settings. The CDC emphasized the need for all professionals to consider all patients potentially infected with HIV-1, other blood-borne pathogens, or both. They further recommended rigorous adherence to infection-control precautions for minimizing the risk of exposure to blood and body fluids of all patients. Salient points for SLPs and audiologists include:

1. Gloves should be worn when touching body fluids, mucous membranes, or nonintact skin of all patients (such as could occur during

an oral-peripheral exam); when handling surfaces soiled with such fluids; and when performing invasive procedures (such as fiberoptic endoscope, tracheostomy tubes, or tracheal-esophageal puncture accessories).

2. Care must be used in the sterilization of instruments. Examples would include tympanometer and otoscope tips, hearing aids (because of contact with cerumen), and flexible endoscopic accessories. The use of a sporocidal chemical is recommended for sterilization of instruments that are used in invasive procedures. Intermediate level disinfection is suggested for other instruments used in noninvasive procedures.

3. Clinicians with nonintact skin, such as from dermatitis, cuts, and the like, should refrain from direct patient care or the handling of contaminated materials. (If the skin is not intact and the clinician must do any touching of the patient, double gloving is recommended.)

Since the emergence of AIDS, the routine use of latex gloves as well as other latex products has increased greatly. With this increased use of latex, a significant prevalence of latex-related allergies, including life-threatening anaphylaxis, has emerged (Berky, Luciano, & James, 1992). **Anaphylaxis** is an allergic hypersensitivity reaction of the body to a foreign substance. If an allergy to latex is developed, it could result in anaphylactic shock, and death may occur if emergency medical treatment is not given.

Although vinyl gloves could be worn instead of latex, latex gloves appear to be preferable as a barrier to HIV-1 (Weiss, 1997). Further research is needed to determine risk reduction and efficacy of using vinyl gloves given the significant and increasing prevalence of latex reactions.

Management of Occupationally Exposed Persons

Little information is available with which to develop the most effective strategy for managing occupational exposures to HIV-1. However, HIV-1 is a fragile virus and the literature suggests that simply washing the cutaneous site of exposure with soap and water is the most appropriate approach. The use of bleach or other disinfecting agents has not been shown to be more efficacious than cleaning with soap and water alone (Osguthorpe, 1992). Mucous membrane splashes with material that might contain HIV should be flushed or rinsed with sterile water or eye irrigant. If none is available, clean tap water is an acceptable alternative.

Individuals who have been occupationally exposed to HIV-1 have the option to undergo experimental postexposure treatment involving reverse transcriptase inhibitors such as the drug zidovudine (AZT). Although reverse transcriptase inhibitors do not prevent HIV-1 from entering cells, it is hoped that the drug will significantly decrease the number of HIV-1 produced by replication. The study that led to this hypothesis (CDC, 1994) demonstrated that AZT treatment of a selected cohort of pregnant women and their newborns was associated with a 68% reduction in perinatal transmission, as compared with the rate among untreated pairs of mothers and infants.

With the widespread availability of AZT as a licensed antiretroviral agent, this postexposure option has gained in popularity although there has been no documentation about the efficacy of treatment. The single most important aspect of AZT or other reverse transcriptase inhibitor therapy is prompt administration of the drug as soon after exposure as possible. Animal studies strongly suggest that delayed treatment, especially beyond 24 hours, is much less beneficial (CDC, 1990). The individual remains on an AZT regimen for 4 to 6 weeks. A liver function test and blood tests are accomplished every 2 weeks to assess any side effects to the prophylactic regimen.

Reverse transcriptase inhibitors cause documented side effects that vary in severity from person to person. These side effects include nausea, fatigue, insomnia, and headaches. There is increased prevalence of drug resistance with early treatment (Gerberding, 1995; Weiss, 1997) that may limit options in treatment later in the course of the disease. There are special concerns due to drug toxicity, including concerns about potential for mutagenicity (genetic mutation) and carcinogenicity (origin of cancers) in the future.

In late 1995, the CDC studied the impact of AZT as a protection against seroconversion in occupationally exposed health care workers. The study was inconclusive as to the value of AZT therapy after exposure. Because there are several known possible side effects to taking AZT (discussed in the previous paragraph), zidovudine benefits do not clearly outweigh the risks of exposure. In the absence of demonstration of high clinical efficacy in the postexposure setting and with the many potential side effects, physicians are hesitant to recommend its use. Therefore, the decision to use postexposure prophylaxis is a difficult one.

The time period following an occupational exposure is a difficult one psychologically for the exposed person (Gerberding, 1995). Reassurance of the low statistical risk of acquisition of a lethal infection may be insufficient at this time. Referral to mental health professionals for crisis management or ongoing stress management may be required.

CHAPTER SUMMARY

Clinical management of clients with HIV-1 infection presents unique challenges. In the past, referral for services from communication disorders professionals did not occur until the end stages of AIDS. Due to the growing success of drug interventions in prolonging the life of those with HIV-1 infection, trends in their care have changed. HIV-1 is a multisystemic disease and requires a multi- and interdisciplinary team approach to effectively provide quality care.

The communication and swallowing impairments associated with HIV-1 frequently are neurogenic in nature. Even during early stages of infection, when no overt signs of disease progression are evident, there is subtle damage occurring in the CNS. For this reason, SLPs and audiologists should participate in the initial evaluation process. Education of other healthcare professional and the public is needed in order to increase earlier referrals.

One of the challenges of working with clients with HIV-1 infection is the fear of contracting the deadly disease from the clients. Although the risk of HIV-1 transmission to SLPs and audiologists is relatively small, precautions must be taken in the clinical setting. To minimize risk of occupational exposure, all clinicians should be knowledgeable about the nature of HIV-1 infection, its signs and symptoms, and strategies to diminish the incidence of skin and mucous exposure of bodily fluids and secretions.

 **4**

Central
Nervous System
Manifestations

In the United States, neurologic disease is recorded for as many as 100,000 people annually infected with HIV-1 (Simpson & Berger, 1996). The nervous system is among the most frequent and serious targets of HIV-1 infection. CNS involvement frequently is both debilitating and life-threatening. Autopsy studies have revealed CNS abnormalities in 80 to 100% of HIV-1-infected adults in the United States and elsewhere (Chimelli, Rosember, Hahn, Lope, & Barretto Netto, 1992; Gray et al., 1993).

Although CNS involvement can occur at any stage of infection, the majority of clinical attention and research has focused on the late stages of HIV-1 infection. Generally, the most aggressive and severe neurologic pathologies are associated with later stages of the disease. However, HIV-1 infection can be accompanied by clinically significant neurologic disorders as early as the time of initial systemic infection. In 10 to 20% of seropositive individuals, neurologic disease is the initial presenting feature (Mehta & Kula, 1992; Simpson & Berger, 1996). In 6% of individuals infected with HIV-1, it may be the only manifestation (Mehta & Kula, 1992).

The difference in the rate of clinically detected neurologic disease and that recorded in autopsy studies may occur because neurologic abnormalities are often overlooked when they coexist with other life-threatening systemic disorders. Careful neurologic examination, even in the absence of specific complaints, frequently reveals evidence of central or peripheral nervous system dysfunction.

RESEARCH INTO CNS PATHOLOGIES
ASSOCIATED WITH HIV-1

The majority of research into neurologic pathologies and their correspond-
ing incidence data, sites of lesion, and clinical manifestations was
undertaken in the early- to mid-1980s. Vast documentation of the effect
of HIV-1 on the CNS was achieved early and the accuracy of that data has
been supported by repeated studies over the years.

Medical and scientific research in the 1990s primarily centered on HIV
itself: advances in knowledge about its genome and applying that knowledge to assess drug effect on virus physiology. Relatively few studies on
HIV-1-related CNS disorders were published between 1991 to 1997. These
recent studies have generally corroborated the data of the earlier findings.

The more recent data show increased incidence of many systemic
pathologies. This increase is due to advances made in detecting the pathology using recently developed biomedical technology. In addition,
healthcare professionals' increased awareness of HIV-1 infection has resulted in more reporting of these data to authorities. Another reason for
the statistical increase is that patients with HIV-1 infection are living
longer due to the drug therapies readily available. However, prolonging
life in an immunosupressed state has resulted in increased incidence of
many systemic pathologies, including those of the CNS.

In the next section, a description of each of the common CNS disorders associated with HIV-1 infection is presented. The known incidence
rates, sites of lesion, and other salient features of each pathology will be
discussed. Tables 4–1 and 4–2 present summaries of the HIV-1-related
CNS disorders categorized in the setting of HIV-1 disease.

As shown in Table 4–2, the disorders are divided into four general
categories: (1) primary infection of the CNS by HIV-1; (2) secondary infection of the CNS by opportunistic infections (via parasitic, fungal, viral, and
bacterial organisms); (3) secondary effect on the CNS by neoplasms; and
(4) secondary CNS complications via HIV-associated systemic disorders.

PRIMARY INFECTION OF THE CNS BY HIV-1

AIDS Dementia

HIV-1 can infect the CNS directly. The most common CNS illness associated with HIV-1 is variously called AIDS dementia complex (ADC),
HIV-1 encephalitis, AIDS encephalopathy, and HIV cognitive-motor complex. The term ADC will be used in this discussion.

ADC is one of the most significant complications associated with
HIV-1 infection. Most published studies and textbooks estimate that

Table 4–1. Major HIV-1-related central nervous system disorders in adults.

CNS Structure	Incidence
Brain	
PREDOMINANTLY NONFOCAL	
Common	
AIDS dementia complex	33–90%
Cytomegalovirus (CMV) encephalitis	15–33%
Metabolic encephalitis	19%
Toxoplasmosis (encephalitic form)	3–40%
Uncommon	
Aspergillosis	4.6%
PREDOMINANTLY FOCAL	
Common	
Cerebral toxoplasmosis	2–15%
Herpes simplex ventriculitis	2%
Infarction	19–20%
Primary central nervous system lymphoma (PCNSL)	3–10%
Progressive multifocal leukoencephalopathy (PML)	2–5%
Varicella-zoster virus encephalitis	0.8–2%
Cryptococcal infection	2.6–13.3%
Mycobacterium avium intracellulare	28.3%
MENINGES	
Common	
Aseptic meningitis	7%
Cryptococcal meningitis	5–12%
Uncommon	
Coccidioidomycosis	<1%
Histoplasmosis	0.7%
Mycobacterium tuberculosis (tuberculous meningitis)	<1%
Syphilitic meningitis	<1%
SPINAL CORD	
Common	
Vacuolar myelopathy	20–30%
Uncommon	
Cytomegalovirus myelopathy	unknown
HTLV-I-associated myelopathy	unknown
Spinal epidural or intradural lymphoma	unknown
Varicella-zoster virus myelopathy	unknown

Source: From "Associated communications disorders and dysphagia in adults with HIV-1 and secondary CNS lesions" by C. R. Larsen, 1996, p. 47. Unpublished master's independent study, University of North Dakota, Grand Forks.

Table 4–2. Common CNS disorders in the setting of HIV-1 disease.

Primary Infection by HIV-1
AIDS dementia complex (HIV encephalopathy)
Aseptic meningitis/Isolated headache
Vacuolar myelopathy

Opportunistic Infections
Cytomegalovirus (CMV)
Fungal encephalitis (meningoencephalitis, aspergillosis, coccidioidomycosis)
Neurosyphilis
Progressive multifocal leukoencephalopathy (PML)
Toxoplasma encephalitis (toxoplasmosis)
Tuberculosis meningitis

CNS Neoplasms
Primary CNS lymphoma (PCNSL)
Non-Hodgkin's lymphoma
Kaposi's sarcoma

Systemic Disorders
Metabolic and Nutritional Diseases
Anemia
Hypoglycemia
Hyponatremia
Hypoxemia
Uremia
Vitamin B12 deficiency

Cerebrovascular Disorders
Infarcts
Intracerebral or subarachnoid hemorrhage
Strokes
Subdural hematoma
Transient ischemic attacks

---

between 28.2% and 66% of people with AIDS eventually will develop moderate to substantial dementia, and another 25% will develop mild dementia (Greenwood, 1991; Petito, Cho, Lemann, Navia, & Price, 1986). One group of researchers found that as many as 90 of their 100 study subjects with AIDS had dementia (Price et al., 1988; Price et al., 1992). However, a few studies have found a low prevalence of neuropsychological deficits until the most advanced stages of HIV-1 infection (McArthur et al., 1989; Miller et al., 1990).

In some cases, ADC may be the presenting or sole manifestation of HIV-1 infection. The syndrome is characterized by initial cognition impairment followed by progressive dementia (Greenwood, 1991). The early clinical picture of ADC resembles depression (Holland & Tross, 1985).

Typical initial symptoms include forgetfulness and poor concentration. Psychomotor retardation, decreased alertness, apathy, social withdrawal, diminished interest in work, and loss of sex drive develop soon after. This often is accompanied by fever or mild metabolic derangement (Price et al., 1988; Price et al., 1992). Less commonly, individuals demonstrate facial nerve paralysis (21.7%) (Belec et al., 1988), motor weakness (34%), personality change (38%), or transient dysarthrias or movement disorders (7%) (Navia, Jordan, & Price, 1986). R. W. Price and associates have carefully studied the clinical profile of patients with ADC and coined the term **AIDS dementia complex.** Table 4–3 presents a summary of their findings.

With advancing dementia, new learning and memory deteriorate. Consequently, there is a further slowing of mental processing, and language impairment becomes more evident. The terminal phases of the syndrome are characterized by a global impairment. Over several months, increased confusion, disorientation, seizures, mutism, profound dementia, coma, and death ensue. The progression of symptoms may occur extremely rapidly over a period of a few weeks, but more typically the decline occurs over several months (Holland & Tross, 1985).

Table 4–3. Symptoms of AIDS-related dementia.

Early Stage Symptoms
Cognition
  Impaired concentration
  Forgetfulness
  Slowing of mental processes
Motor
  Unsteady gait
  Leg weakness
  Loss of coordination, impaired handwriting
  Tremor
Behavior
  Apathy, withdrawal, personality change
  Agitation, confusion, hallucinations
Late Stage Symptoms
Mental Status
  Global dementia
  Psychomotor slowing: verbal responses delayed, progressive mutism,
    vacant stare
  Unaware of illness or deficits, disinhibition
  Confusion, disorientation
  Organic psychosis

In late stage ADC, incontinence may be prominent and the incidence of ataxia, motor weakness, and tremors increases (Price et al., 1988; Price et al., 1992). Increased tone development that often is associated with tremor, clonus (spasmodic alternation of muscular contraction and relaxation), and hyperactive reflexes, particularly in the lower extremities, have been noted in some individuals with HIV-1 infection. This condition may reflect the effects of an accompanying HIV-related myelopathy. Without treatment, the dementia is rapidly progressive, with mean survival of about 6 months. There currently is no effective therapy for ADC.

Hearing loss in ADC has been reported (Hart et al., 1989). Involvement of the inferior colliculus may explain the central auditory dysfunction associated with subacute encephalitis. Auditory brainstem response (ABR) findings in individuals with AIDS are consistent with a central demyelinating disorder.

Aseptic Meningitis and Isolated Headache

Aseptic meningitis is a syndrome related to direct HIV-1 infection of the leptomeninges. It may occur at the time of acute HIV-1 infection, but is more common in individuals with advanced infection. Hollander and Stringari (1987) divided the disorder into two types: an acute form and a chronic form. Both are accompanied by meningeal symptoms, such as headaches and photophobia (intolerance to light). However, meningeal signs such as nuchal rigidity (stiff neck) are mostly characteristic of the acute form of meningitis. Cranial nerve palsies may also be a complication, particularly affecting cranial nerves V, VII, or VIII, with Bell's palsy sometimes occurring.

Isolated headache is a common symptom and occurs in the same clinical setting as aseptic meningitis. The cause of this type of headache is uncertain, but the pain can be severe and intractable. In some individuals, it appears to relate to development of systemic disease and may be caused by metabolic imbalance and production of certain toxins.

Vacuolar Myelopathy

In early 1985, vacuolar myelopathy, a unique HIV-related central neurological syndrome, was first described (Petito et al., 1985). The infection involves the demyelination of the spinal column. The demyelination of the white matter of the spinal cord is especially concentrated in the posterior and lateral white columns of the thoracic spinal cord (Petito et al., 1985). Autopsy studies have demonstrated the disorder in 20 to 33% of random patients with AIDS (Petito et al., 1985; Petito, Vecchio, & Chen, 1994).

The most common symptoms associated with vacuolar myelopathy include leg weakness, spasticity, gait disorders, and incontinence. Neurological examination often reveals paraparesis (partial paralysis affecting the lower limbs), spasticity (increased tone or contractions of muscles causing stiff and awkward movements), and ataxia (deficit in coordinating voluntary muscle control). Vacuolar myelopathy often accompanies AIDS dementia complex.

SECONDARY INFECTION OF THE CNS BY OPPORTUNISTIC INFECTIONS

The previous section discussed how primary infection of the CNS occurs when there is direct infection of the nervous system by HIV-1. However, secondary infection of the CNS occurs when HIV-1 infects another system in the body through an opportunistic infection, neoplasm, or systemic disorder initially and then is disseminated to the nervous system.

Opportunistic infections are infections caused by any organism, but especially parasitic, fungal, and bacterial. Infection occurs due to the opportunity afforded by the altered physiological state of the host. HIV-1 causes immune suppression in the infected person, allowing certain microorganisms that otherwise would be nonpathogenic to become pathogenic.

Neoplasms are new and abnormal formations of tissue, such as a growth or tumor. They serve no beneficial function and grow at the expense of surrounding healthy tissue. The neoplasm may metastasize, or spread from one part of the body to another. The metastasis may occur via a lymph vessel or bloodstream.

Some patients with HIV-1 infection exhibit transient neurologic deficits that are unrelated to an underlying opportunistic infection or neoplasm. Secondary CNS complications may occur due to HIV-1-associated systemic disorders. The most common systemic disorders associated with HIV-1 infection are cerebrovascular pathologies or metabolic diseases. The following section will describe opportunistic infections, neoplasms, and systemic disorders that may result in secondary infection of the CNS.

Common Parasitic Infection

Cerebral Toxoplasmosis

Toxoplasma gondii, an intracellular protozoan, is among the most prevalent causes of latent infection of the CNS throughout the world (American Foundation for AIDS Research, 1995). Infection occurs primarily via the oral route through ingestion of raw or undercooked meat. The parasite is so common that more than half of all adults in the United States have been infected with the parasite. It rarely causes disease in persons whose immune system is intact. The *Toxoplasma gondii* organism remains in the body tissues as cysts that do not multiply and do not cause disease. Once the immune system of an individual becomes compromised, the dormant organisms may become reactivated. Most toxoplasmosis in HIV-1 infection is the result of reactivation of old infection, and the brain is the most common site of involvement.

Toxoplasmosis is the most frequent of the HIV-1-associated opportunistic infections. The reported incidence of toxoplasmosis ranges from 3 to 40% (Petito et al., 1986; Porter & Sande, 1992; Vinters & Anders, 1990). Thrombosis (development or existence of a blood clot in the vascular system) of blood vessels causing large areas of coagulation necrosis may produce multiple mass lesions in the brain. The lesions are most commonly bilateral and involve the cerebral cortex (near the gray-white junction) and deep gray nuclei (basal ganglia). Multiple lesions are located in the frontal, basal ganglia, and parietal regions (Porter & Sande, 1992). Less commonly, the cerebellum, brainstem, or spinal cord are involved (Vinters & Anders, 1990).

Cerebral toxoplasmosis is generally subacute, evolving over several days from initial symptoms to presentation with neurologic deficit. Focal cerebral dysfunction usually predominate but often is combined with diffuse signs and symptoms. In a retrospective review, Porter and Sande (1992) described their experience with toxoplasmosis of the CNS in 115 adult patients with HIV-1 infection at San Francisco General Hospital. The most common presenting symptoms were headache (55%), confusion (52%), fever (47%), lethargy (43%), and seizures (29%). Focal neurological abnormalities included hemiparesis (39%), ataxia (30%), cranial nerve palsies (28%), aphasia (8%), and visual field deficit (7%). Movement disorders, such as poor coordination, gait disturbance, and focal weakness, were seen in approximately 25% of the cases.

Another study of toxoplasmic encephalitis was carried out by Luft and associates (1993). Neurologic assessment of 49 study subjects included an evaluation of 26 signs and symptoms. The assessment was divided into five neuroanatomical categories: diffuse cortical; nonlocalizing; subcortical or cerebellar; focal cortical; and brainstem, cord, or peripheral. At baseline, more than 50% of the subjects had abnormalities in three categories: subcortical and cerebellar, focal cortical, and nonlocalizing.

Common Fungal Infections

Cryptococcal Meningitis

Cryptococcus neoformans is a yeast-like fungus that is found worldwide, particularly in soil contaminated with bird excrement (American Foundation for AIDS Research, 1995). This fungus is the most common cause of fungal infection of the CNS in HIV-1-infected individuals and has been reported at 2.6 to 3.3% in one autopsy study (Petito et al., 1986) and 5 to 12% in another clinical and autopsy study (Vinters & Anders, 1990). The tissue damage characteristic of fungal meningoencephalitis caused by *Cryptococcus* is generally the same in individuals with or without HIV-1 infection, except that in cases of immunosuppression, the damage is more extensive and destructive. Individuals with crytococcal infection of the CNS have chronic meningitis with abnormalities of the cerebrospinal fluid (CSF). This typically affects the leptomeninges (pia mater and arachnoid), which become thickened by reactive connective tissue (De Girolami & Smith, 1992). This thickened tissue may impede the flow of CSF from the foramina of Luschka and Magendie, giving rise to hydrocephalus (increased accumulation of CSF within the ventricles of the brain).

Cryptococcal meningitis most frequently manifests as a subacute meningitis with symptoms that include headache, nausea, fever, vomiting, seizure, fatigue, stiff neck, and confusion. Fever and headache are the most common features of infection. Facial nerve paralysis has been reported in 8.7% of individuals with Cryptococcus infection (Belec et al., 1988).

Sensorineural hearing loss is associated with infection by *Cryptococcus neoformans* in 27% of patients and may be sudden or progressive (Lewis & Rabinovich, 1972). Temporal bone findings include infiltration of the cochlear nerve, vestibular nerve, and Scarpa's ganglion with cryptococcal organisms, microphages (a small phagocyte or cell that is able to ingest and destroy particulate substances such as bacteria and cells), and exudates with early necrosis of the nerve (McGill, 1978). Additional temporal bone pathology includes edematous stria vascularis and mild endolymphatic hydrops involving the cochlea and the saccule. Peripheral end organ damage with necrosis of the organ of Corti in the cochlea, epithelium of the otolithic organs, and the semicircular canal have also been noted (Kwartler, Linthicum, Jahn, & Hawke, 1991). Cryptococcal infection often is complicated by frequent recurrences.

Other Fungal Infections

Candida albicans is a yeastlike fungi that reproduces by budding. Commonly part of the normal flora of the mouth, skin, intestinal tract, and vagina, the fungi is kept under control by an intact immune system. However, when immunosuppression occurs, the fungi is given opportunity to grow out of control, resulting in infection. *Candida albicans* is the most frequent cause of esophageal pathogen in HIV disease. The common complaint with esophageal candidiasis is diffuse odynophagia (pain or discomfort during swallowing), dysphagia, or both (Friedman, 1994). Less frequently, *Candida albicans* also can infect the CNS and cause meningoencephalitis (Levy & Berger, 1992). The incidence of *Candida* infection of the CNS has been reported at 1.3 to 19.7% (Petito et al., 1986).

Common Viral Infections

Cytomegalovirus (CMV)

Cytomegalovirus (CMV) is the most common opportunistic viral pathogen affecting the CNS. Evidence of prior exposure to CMV is present in approximately 80% of adults over age 40 and in higher rates among homosexuals (Mehta & Kula, 1992). CMV is a DNA herpes virus that becomes latent after primary infection, and reactivation occurs only in association with immune dysfunction. In the pre-AIDS era, it was seen rarely as a cause of neurologic disease in adults. Now CMV is second only to HIV-1 in producing CNS involvement in AIDS.

Evidence of CMV infection has been noted in 15 to 33% of individuals with HIV-1 infection (American Foundation for AIDS Research, 1995; Petite et al., 1994; Price et al., 1992). The diagnosis of CMV infection is difficult to make without a brain biopsy because it is clinically and radiologically indistinguishable from AIDS dementia complex (ADC). These conditions frequently coexist.

CMV infection can have several different manifestations. The most common pattern of involvement is subacute encephalitis with the formation of microglial nodules primarily within gray matter. The virus tends to localize in the ependyma (membrane lining the cerebral ventricles) and subependymal regions of the brain. This can result in severe necrotizing ventriculoencephalitis with massive necrosis (death of an area of tissue surrounded by healthy tissue), hemorrhage, ventriculitis (inflammation of a ventricle), and choroid plexitis (inflammation of the choroid plexus). Facial nerve palsy has been noted in nearly 11% of subjects infected with CMV in one study (Belec et al., 1988).

Systemic CMV infection—retinal, gastrointestinal, and pulmonary— is very common in HIV-1 infection. CMV infection of the gastrointestinal system can cause esophagitis that leads to severe odynophagia and some dysphagia (Friedman, 1994). Like CMV infection in other systems, esophageal disease generally is confined to late-stage HIV-1 infection.

Herpes Simplex Virus (HSV)

Herpes simplex virus (HSV) is a common cause of encephalitis in normal hosts and has been associated with HIV-1 infection of the CNS. There are two forms of HSV: HSV-1 and HSV-2. HSV-1 is the usual cause of encephalitis in adults, which occurs from reactivation of the dormant virus in cranial nerve ganglia acquired during childhood. Prior to the advent of HIV-1, HSV-2 produced encephalitis only in the newborn period. Now, it also can be acquired by adults through sexual contact, becoming latent in the sacral ganglia, and may give rise to aseptic meningitis on reactivation when the immune system is compromised (Mehta & Kula, 1992). The incidence of HSV infection was reported at 2.0% in a neuropathologic study of 153 adult subjects by Petito and associates (1986). Other significant findings about HSV of interest to SLPs and audiologists include:

- Facial nerve palsy reported in approximately 11% of individuals with HIV-1 infection and HSV (Belec et al., 1988)
- Dysphagia associated with HSV infection (Friedman, 1994)
- Sudden hearing loss (Wilson, 1986)

Varicella Zoster Virus (VZV)

Varicella zoster virus (VZV), which causes chicken pox in children and zoster (shingles) in adults, is associated with several neurologic syndromes. These include encephalitis, leukoencephalopathy, cerebritis (inflammation of the cerebrum), cranial neuropathies, aseptic meningitis, cerebral vasculitis, myelitis (inflammation of the spinal cord or bone marrow), and radiculitis (inflammation of spinal nerve roots) (Mehta & Kula, 1992).

VZV encephalitis is uncommon, seen in only 0.8 to 2% of autopsied individuals with HIV-1 infection (Levy, Bredesen, & Rosenblum, 1985; Petito et al., 1986). Lesions are in both the white and gray matter. Multifocal lesions in the white matter with demyelination and thrombosis of vessels often are seen together. Sudden sensorineural hearing loss also has been documented (Wilson, 1986).

Progressive Multifocal Leukoencephalopathy (PML)

Progressive multifocal leukoencephalopathy (PML) is a progressive demyelinating disease of the central nervous system that is opportunistic in immune-compromised individuals. PML is caused by the activation of a common papovavirus (a group of viruses important in causing viral-related cancer), the J. C. virus (JCV). JCV infects oligodendrocytes in the brain that produce myelin, a vital substance that protects axons (a process of a neuron that conducts impulses away from the cell body).

Approximately 70% of all adults in the United States have antibodies to JCV, indicating prior infection. Most cases of PML are believed to be due to reactivation of latent JCV infection in individuals whose immune system becomes compromised. Inactive or latent JCV is harbored in the kidneys. When the immune system malfunctions, β lymphocytes transport

JCV to the brain from bone marrow. The incidence of PML in individuals infected with HIV-1 is 2 to 5% (American Foundation for AIDS Research, 1995; Petito et al., 1986; Levy et al., 1985).

PML is characterized by selective demyelination, most often in the subcortical white matter. Pathologic examination of the lesions shows patchy, ill-defined granular destruction of the white matter ranging in size from a few millimeters to involvement of an entire lobe of the brain, cerebellar hemisphere, or brainstem (Price et al., 1992). Lesions generally begin as small loci and then coalesce to form larger lesions.

Onset of PML is subacute and evolves over weeks (Worley & Price, 1992). PML presents with mild cognitive or behavioral changes, followed by focal (starting point of a disease process) neurologic deficits that become progressively worse. These include hemiparesis (paralysis affecting one half of the body), hemianopia (blindness for half the visual field in one or both eyes), hemisensory deficit, ataxia (deficits in coordinating voluntary muscle movements), altered mental status, personality changes, and speech or language deficits (American Foundation for AIDS Research, 1995; Mehta & Kula, 1992; Price et al., 1992). There is also evidence that PML is associated with profound hearing loss (Wilson, 1986).

Common Bacterial Infection

Neurosyphilis

Neurosyphilis is a form of syphilis that infects the nervous system. There is some evidence that suggests that HIV-1 may alter the natural course of neurosyphilis, and that meningovascular syphilis (a form of neurosyphilis that involves the meninges and vascular structures in the brain or spinal cord or both) and otosyphilis (a form of neurosyphilis that affects the inner ear) may occur more commonly and earlier in those with HIV-1 infection. CNS involvement by syphilis may be manifest as asymptomatic infection, acute syphilitic meningitis, cerebral arthritis, stroke, deafness, as well as optic neuropathy (such as eye inflammation and swollen or damaged retinas) (Gordon et al., 1994).

The rate of progression and severity of neurosyphilis and otosyphilis appear to follow an accelerated rate in patients with HIV-1 infection. In patients with HIV-1 infection, the interval between primary infection by syphilis and manifestation of otosyphilis is shortened from the typical 15 to 30 years to 2 to 5 years (Smith & Canalis, 1989). CNS involvement by syphilis may be manifested as asymptomatic infection, acute syphilitic meningitis, cerebral arthritis, stroke, optic neuropathy (such as eye inflammation and swollen or damaged retinas), and deafness (Gordon et al., 1994). Diagnosis of otosyphilis is supported by a suggestive clinical history, unilateral or bilateral sensorineural low-frequency hearing loss, and hydropic labyrinthine symptoms. Stabilization or improvement of hearing and speech discrimination with penicillin and steroid treatment further supports the diagnosis of otosyphilis (Gordon et al, 1994; Smith & Canalis, 1989).

OPPORTUNISTIC CNS LYMPHOMAS

Lymphoma, or neoplasm, is a growth of new tissue, benign or malignant, in the lymphatic system. The risk of developing CNS lymphoma in the general population has been estimated at 0.0001% (Berry, Hooton, Collier, & Lukehart, 1987). In the HIV-1-infected population, the risk is approximately 2%. The annual incidence of primary CNS lymphoma (PCNSL) in the United States prior to the AIDS epidemic was 225 cases. In 1986, an estimated 240 cases were reported. By 1991, more than 1800 cases occurred, indicating that PCNSL is a disease predominantly affecting the AIDS patient population (Levy et al., 1989).

Primary CNS lymphoma affects the CNS by developing directly in the brain or spinal cord. In contrast, opportunistic lymphomas can affect the CNS through secondary infection by metastasis to the central nervous system (CNS) from other sites. Metastatic or secondary CNS lymphoma has been reported with greater frequency (Auperin et al., 1994; Levy et al., 1989).

Primary CNS Lymphoma (PCNSL)

Primary central nervous system lymphoma (PCNSL) is second only to toxoplasmosis as a cause of focal cerebral masses in AIDS (Levy & Berger, 1992). PCNSL more frequently involves the brain parenchyma (the functional parts of the brain such as the white matter and gray matter) (Levy & Berger, 1992). Autopsy data show that the incidence of PCNSL is 3 to 10% in individuals with HIV-1 infection (Petito et al., 1986; Price et al., 1992). PCNSL generally occurs in the late stages of HIV-1 infection (Price et al., 1992; Simpson & Berger, 1996).

Researchers have detected the presence of Epstein-Barr virus (believed to be he causative agent in infectious mononucleosis) in PCNSL with an incidence approaching 100% (Auperin et al., 1994; Simpson & Berger, 1996). A common manifestation of PCNSL is encephalopathy followed by cranial polyneuropathy (any noninflammatory disorder of peripheral nerves). The most frequent symptoms are headaches, localized weakness, speech problems, lethargy, and personality changes, which can mimic AIDS dementia complex (ADC). Focal deficits, such as hemiparesis, hemisensory loss, ataxia, and aphasia may be seen (Levy et al., 1989). Less commonly, seizures may occur. One study reported an associated incidence of facial nerve paralysis at 13% (Belec et al., 1988). Sensorineural hearing loss has been associated with PCNSL and other metastic neoplasms (Lalwani & Sooy, 1992).

Systemic Lymphoma with CNS Involvement

Systemic lymphoma complicating HIV-1 infection may involve the CNS secondarily, with an incidence as high as 49% (Price et al., 1992). In contrast to PCNSL, systemic lymphomas often occur early in HIV-1 infection. Another difference between primary and secondary CNS lymphoma is that secondary lymphoma affects the CNS by invasion of the **meninges** (the three membranes lining the spinal cord and brain: dura mater, arachnoid, and pia mater). AIDS-associated lymphoma frequently is metastasized to the CNS by non-Hodgkin's lymphoma (Auperin, 1994).

The initial symptoms of non-Hodgkin's lymphoma include altered cognitive function, cranial nerve palsies, headaches, spinal epidural compression, fever, or night sweats in conjunction with painless enlargement of a lymph node in one part of the body. Lymph nodes in other parts of the body remain unchanged. Because systemic lymphomas occur early in HIV-1 disease, patients tolerate aggressive chemotherapy treatment more easily because they are less medically compromised (Price et al., 1992).

HIV-1-ASSOCIATED SYSTEMIC DISORDERS

Cerebrovascular Complications

Increased incidence of cerebrovascular disease has been found in association with HIV-1 infection; up to a 100-fold increase as compared with age-matched controls has been reported (Levy & Bredesen, 1988). The incidence of cerebrovascular complication in persons with HIV-1 infection has been reported at 19 to 20% (Engstrom, Lowenstein, & Bredesen, 1989; Petito et al., 1986).

Transient ischemic attacks (TIAs), small or large bland or hemorrhagic infarcts, intracerebral or subarachnoid hemorrhage, and subdural hematoma (a swelling or mass of blood located beneath the dura mater) have all been reported in this population (Engstrom et al., 1989). Most ischemic infarcts are small, often multiple, and can be seen in any area of the brain. There is evidence that a vasculopathy (any disease of the blood vessels) associated with an underlying opportunistic process in HIV-1 infection may lead to vascular abnormalities and subsequent stroke in individuals with HIV-1 infection (Kieburtz, Eskin, Ketonen, & Tuite, 1993).

Metabolic and Nutritional Disorders

The rapidly progressive nature of malnutrition appears to be unique to HIV-1. Weight loss is nearly universal in prevalence (Chelbowski et al., 1989), and the term *wasting syndrome* has been used to describe the condition. Multisystemic disorders associated with HIV-1 infection contribute to metabolic and nutritional imbalance. Examples of systemic disorders associated with CNS signs and symptoms include hypoxemia (insufficient oxygenation of the blood), anemia, hyponatremia (decreased concentration of sodium in the blood), hypoglycemia (deficiency of glucose in the blood), uremia (toxic condition associated with renal insufficiency). Other complications that have been described include new onset diabetes mellitus and hyperglycemia (increase of blood sugar as in diabetes) (FDA, 1997), altered lipid (fat or fat-like substance) metabolism (having too much fat or cholesterol in the blood) (Hengel, Watts, & Lennox, 1997), and body composition changes (losing lean mass and increasing percentage of body fat) (Ruane, 1997).

The most common nutritional deficiency in HIV-1-infected individuals is vitamin B12 deficiency and is revealed in 25 % of all AIDS cases (Beach et al., 1992; Petito et al., 1994). Vitamin B12 deficiency leads to **pernicious anemia,** which is a severe form of blood disease characterized by progressive decrease in red blood corpuscles, muscular weakness, and gastrointestinal and neural disturbances. This condition may be fatal if not treated with vitamin B12, iron, and diet. Symptoms include weakness, sore tongue, tingling and numbness of extremities, and gastrointestinal symptoms such as diarrhea, nausea, vomiting, and pain. In severe pernicious anemia, signs of cardiac failure may be present.

As individuals with HIV-1 disease survive longer, the impact of recurrent and chronic infections on cognitive function and nutrition becomes more relevant to their overall care. HIV-1 disease, immune function, enteric (digestive system) infection, malnutrition, and malabsorption are interrelated. When a person becomes malnourished secondary to malabsorption following an enteric infection, the immune system declines, predisposing that individual to other infections which then further increases the risk of progressive malnutrition.

Multisystemic illnesses contribute to a number of metabolic and nutritional brain disorders in individuals with HIV-1 infection. These disorders include:

- encephalopathies (brain dysfunction) related to hypoxemia (Price et al., 1992),
- toxic encephalopathies (brain dysfunction) due to various medications with CNS side effects (Price et al., 1992),
- neuropsychological changes associated with vitamin B12 deficiency (Petito et al., 1994),

- deficits of extrapyramidal motor systems (i.e., spasticity, tremors, impaired muscle tone) related to drug therapy (Hollander et al., 1985),
- Wernicke's encephalopathy associated with thiamin deficiency (Price et al., 1992), and
- cognitive deficits due to metabolic imbalance secondary to toxic drug therapies.

CHAPTER SUMMARY

The effect of HIV-1 infection on the central nervous system is profound and widespread. Neurologic disease is recorded for as many as 100,000 people annually infected with HIV-1. Autopsy studies have revealed CNS abnormalities in 80 to 100% of HIV-1-infected adults in the United States and elsewhere. As more effective treatments of the disease prolong the lives of infected individuals, the prevalence of neurologic disorders will likely increase.

Central nervous system disorders associated with HIV-1 are many and varied, as are their related signs and symptoms. The differential diagnosis of neurological syndromes is made more difficult because it is not unusual to find multiple HIV-1-related CNS pathologies in one patient. Nearly one third of all brain autopsies reveals the existence of multiple intracranial pathologies (Levy et al., 1989).

At this time, no further elaboration can be made regarding speech, language, hearing, and cognitive dysfunction associated with CNS disorders related to HIV-1 infection in the adult population due to lack of research in the field of communication disorders. The data concerning adults with HIV-1 infection presented here and elsewhere in this book are obtained primarily from the medical field. The information presented in this chapter is meant to serve as a base of knowledge to build on with future research. Chapter 6 presents data on pediatric HIV-1 infection and associated communication disorders.

 **5**

Head and Neck Manifestations, Otologic Manifestations, and Dysphagia Associated with HIV-1 Infection

In addition to the multiple disorders of the central nervous system, HIV-1 is responsible for numerous manifestations of the head and head, neurotologic disorders, and dysphagia. Persons infected with HIV-1 present with a wide spectrum of systemic disorders requiring a multidisciplinary approach to provide the best care. This chapter will discuss the most common complaints in each of these areas and consider the implications they present for a client's ability to communicate, interpret sound, and maintain adequate nutritional status.

HEAD AND NECK MANIFESTATIONS

Head and neck manifestations are common in HIV-1 infection. Initial reports in the late 1980s stated that head and neck manifestations occurred in 40% of the cases (Flower & Sooy, 1987). With the inclusion of new disease entities in the definition of AIDS and increased accuracy of reporting, more recent reports state that nearly 100% of patients with AIDS present with head and neck manifestations during the course of the disease (Dichtel, 1992; Lalwani & Sooy, 1992). Therefore, it is imperative to do a thorough oral-peripheral examination, not only during initial evaluation but intermittently during ongoing therapy.

Head and neck complaints associated with HIV-1 infection include oral manifestations, diseases of the nose and paranasal sinuses, and ophthalmic complications. The majority of the disorders are due to opportunistic infections that occur in the course of HIV-1 disease progression.

Oropharyngeal Manifestations

Many of the complications of HIV-1 infection involve the mouth. This is because the oral cavity normally hosts a multitude of microflora, and an intact immune system is able to maintain a balance so that no fungal, bacterial, or viral infection occurs. However, the person whose immune system is suppressed due to HIV-1 suffers from several systemic and metabolic imbalances that allow the microflora to grow unchecked, causing oral complications. It is particularly important for a person with HIV-1 to exercise good oral hygiene and get regular dental care. Though most complications occur in the later stages of the disease, many individuals exhibit oral complications early.

Oral lesions are often an early manifestation of HIV-1 infection. They can be identified in 40% of all persons infected with HIV-1 and in nearly 100% of persons with AIDS (Battinelli & Peters, 1995; Dichtel, 1992). Therefore, identification of any of these lesions in a patient not previously known to be infected by HIV-1 may suggest the need for HIV testing. If the patient is known to have HIV-1 then the appearance of oral manifestations may signal disease progression toward AIDS (Cruz et al., 1996; Phelan, 1997).

Most oral lesions are caused by fungal, bacterial, or viral agents. Additional causes of complications include neoplasms (such as a tumor or growth) and lesions caused by something other than a fungal, bacterial, or viral agent. Table 5–1 provides a summary of the reported oral manifestations in persons with HIV-1 infection. A brief description of these lesions follows.

Fungal Opportunistic Infections

The most common fungal infection of the mouth is oral candidiasis (Dichtel, 1992; Phelan, 1997). Oral candidiasis is an opportunistic infection that is usually caused by the fungus *Candida albicans,* a fungus which is

Table 5–1. Common oral manifestations in HIV-1 infection.

Fungal	Viral
Candidiasis	Herpes simplex virus
Pseudomembranous	Herpes zoster virus
Erythematous	Hairy leukoplakia
Angular cheilitis	Cytomegalovirus (CMV) ulcers
Hyperplastic	Human papillomavirus (Warts)
Histoplasmosis	**Neoplastic Diseases**
Geotrichosis	Kaposi's sarcoma
Cryptococcosis	Non-Hodgkins's lymphoma
Aspergillosis	Squamous cell carcinoma
Bacterial	**Other Conditions**
HIV-1-associated gingivitis	Recurrent aphthous ulcerations
HIV-1-associated periodontitis	Idiopathic thrombocytopenic
Bacillary epithelioid angiomatosis	purpura
Mycobacterium avium complex	Salivary gland disease/
Necrotizing stomatitis	Xerostomia

found in the mouth of most people. When the fungus grows out of control, candidiasis is the result. This condition can be painless or so severely painful as to interfere with chewing or swallowing.

In HIV-1 infection, the development of oral candidiasis is associated with an increased risk of progression to AIDS or death. It is an important clinical marker in the management of persons with HIV-1. Oral candidiasis is included in the staging system delineated by the Centers for Disease Control and Prevention. The occurrence of oral candidiasis indicates that the immune system is weakening (Bartlett & Finkbeiner, 1993).

Three forms of oral candidiasis are commonly seen in patients with HIV-1 infections: pseudomembranous candidiasis, erythematous candidiasis, and angular cheilitis. **Pseudomembranous candidiasis** is commonly known as *thrush* and can appear on any oral mucosal surface. Symptoms include white or grayish-white patches that look like cottage cheese along the gums, along the inside of the cheeks, or on the tongue. The patches can be scraped off, revealing the red and swollen underlying surface. The scraping may cause bleeding in that area.

Erythematous candidiasis is seen as smooth red patches on the hard or soft palate, buccal mucosa, or dorsal surface of the tongue. These lesions may seem insignificant and may be missed unless a thorough oral examination is undertaken. The red and swollen tissue will generally be sensitive to touch.

Another common form of candidiasis is **angular cheilitis** (disorder of the lip region). This produces red and swollen tissue that cracks, creating ulceration of the corners of the mouth. The area around the affected tissue may also be red.

Reports of *hyperplastic* (excessive tissue) *candidiasis* are more rare than the other three forms. This form appears as thick, curd-like white plaques that cannot be scraped off. The buccal mucosa is the most common site for hyperplastic candidiasis. This form of candidiasis is difficult to distinguish from leukoplakia or hairy leukoplakia. The physician may need to do a biopsy to confirm the diagnosis.

The oral lesions associated with fungal opportunistic infections may cause pain while the person is chewing or swallowing. The ulcerated and swollen mucosal tissue cannot tolerate spicy, very hot, or very cold food and liquids. Soft and bland diet modification can be made to enable the person eat with less pain. Oral candidiasis does not cause pain during swallowing. If the patient is complaining of dysphagia or odynophagia, then the candidiasis may have extended into the esophagus, causing esophagitis. Pharyngeal and esophageal candidiasis frequently accompanies oral candidiasis and may result in significant dysphagia (Dichtel, 1992). The diagnosis of esophagitis can be made by a gastroenterologist using an endoscope or barium swallow.

The fungal infections respond well to both treatment with topical and systemic antifungal agents. However, fungal infections may be persistent and recur despite treatment, and there have been reports of resistant organisms as a result of treatment (Greenspan & Greenspan D, 1995; Phelan, 1997).

Bacterial Opportunistic Infections

Unusual and aggressive forms of **gingivitis** and **periodontitis** (inflammation or degeneration of the gums, alveolar bone, and support of the tooth) are seen in association with HIV-1 infection. HIV-1-related gingivitis is an infection of the gingival margin, gingiva, and occasionally, the alveolar mucosa. The gingiva may show a distinctive inflamed marginal line even in mouths that show little accumulation of plaque. Patients frequently complain of spontaneous bleeding, ulceration or necrosis of the interdental gingiva, and deep, severe pain that is not readily relieved by analgesics. HIV-1-related gingivitis does not respond well to conventional treatment and frequently progresses to HIV-1-related periodontitis.

Periodontal disease occurs in 30 to 50% of AIDS patients (Greenspan, J. S. & Greenspan D., 1995) but is rarely seen in asymptomatic individuals who are HIV positive. The symptoms include linear gingival erythema and ulcerations and soft-tissue necrosis. Rapid destruction of the underlying bone may be observed, with loss of more than 90% of the alveolar bone within a few weeks (Battinelli & Peters, 1993; Phelan, 1997). Untreated periodontitis is rapidly progressive and results in tooth loss.

Gingivitis and periodontitis may involve the entire mouth or they can present as discrete lesions adjacent to areas of healthy tissue (Battinelli & Peters, 1993; Phelan, 1997). There may be rapid progressive loss of gingival and periodontal soft tissues and rapid destruction of supporting bone (Phelan, 1997). Teeth are then at risk of loosening or even falling out.

Treatment for gingivitis and periodontitis that is effective in the general population is not effective in persons with HIV-1 infection. The therapy that is most effective in these cases involves thorough scraping of the oral cavity and debridement (removal of dead or damaged tissue) of diseased hard and soft tissue (Phelan, 1997; Greenspan & Greenspan, 1995). This is followed by application of topical antiseptics and mouthwashes. Treatment will fail if thorough removal of bacteria and necrotized tissue is not achieved and maintained long-term.

Other less frequently occurring bacterial infections of the mouth include bacillary epithelioid angiomatosis, necrotizing stomatitis and *Mycobacterium avium*. **Bacillary epithelioid angiomatosis** is a relatively newly described oral lesion in people with HIV-1 infection (Nevell, Bewley, & Chopra, 1995). The resulting oral lesions are composed of a prominent vascular proliferation, which may resemble Kaposi's sarcoma. These lesions may also appear on the skin. The drug erythromycin is given to fight this infection.

The symptoms of **necrotizing stomatitis** are persistent ulcerations of the soft tissue adjacent to the teeth The infection causes the tissue to die and the destruction involves the bone as well as soft tissue. Some of these lesions respond to debridement and antibiotic therapy.

Mycobacterium avium **complex** infections frequently are seen with AIDS. This bacterial infection usually involves the organs of the mononuclear phagocyte system (lymph node, spleen, liver, marrow). Although it is uncommon to see visible lesions, oral ulcers associated with *Mycobacterium avium* have been reported. Diagnosis requires a culture and medical treatment involves application of topical antibiotics.

Viral Infections

Oral lesions due to herpes simplex virus infection are particularly common in HIV-1 infection. Herpes simplex virus type 1 is the viral strain most commonly involved and infects 9% of AIDS patients (Dichtel, 1992). **Herpes simplex virus** lesions are recurrent intraoral lesions with crops of small, painful vesicles that ulcerate. They commonly appear on the palate or gingiva. The primary infection is characterized by systemic flu-like symptoms accompanied by painful gingival inflammation and multiple oral lesions. The most common recurrent form of herpes simplex virus is called herpes labialis, otherwise known as a cold sore or fever blister.

Herpes simplex infections are more frequent, more severe, and more persistent in people with HIV-1 infection.

The sores usually start as an area of irritation or pain that becomes inflamed, then forms a watery blister that breaks and forms an open sore with pus, and finally scabs over and heals. The sores occur on the lips, in the mouth along the cheeks (buccal mucosa), palate, or on the back of the mouth. It can be painful to eat if the sores are located in a place that is irritated when the person chews. Sores that are in the back of the mouth or esophagus can interfere with swallowing (Bartlett & Finkbeiner, 1993).

When **herpes zoster virus,** which causes shingles, involves the second (maxillary) or third (mandibular) branches of the trigeminal nerve, then orofacial zoster may occur (Battinelli & Peters, 1993). In orofacial zoster, the vesicles and ulcers follow the distribution of one or more branches of the trigeminal nerve on one side, producing unilateral pain. Facial nerve palsy also may occur (Bartlett & Finkbeiner, 1993). The ulcers usually heal in two to three weeks, but pain may persist.

Hairy leukoplakia, which is caused by the Epstein-Barr virus (which is responsible for infectious mononucleosis), was first seen on the tongue in homosexual men in 1984 . This is a common manifestation in people with AIDS, occurring in 5 to 25% of cases (Dichtel, 1992). It was initially believed that hairy leukoplakia was unique to HIV-1 infection but since has been shown to infrequently manifest in other immunosuppressed persons such as kidney, heart, and bone marrow transplant recipients (Greenspan, Greenspan, Pindborg, & Schiodt, 1990). However, almost all patients with hairy leukoplakia are HIV-1 seropositive. The development of the infection signals the subsequent development of AIDS (median time of 24 months from onset of hairy leukoplakia) and death (median time 44 months) (Greenspan & Greenspan, 1995). The severity of the lesions (whether tiny or very extensive) appears not to be relevant in this disease pattern.

Oral hairy leukoplakia is named for its location, in the mouth, and its appearance as white patches (leukoplakia) with microscopic hairlike protrusions from the tongue's surface. The patches can be a fraction of an inch in diameter or they can coat most of the tongue. In addition to the tongue, hairy leukoplakia can cause lesions in buccal mucosa, soft palate, and floor of the mouth. Some people with oral hairy leukoplakia have a sore mouth, which may interfere with eating, and occasionally have voice changes (Bartlett & Finkbeiner, 1993). The usual medical treatment is antiviral drugs taken orally. The patches disappear within a few weeks but the infection frequently recurs when medication is discontinued.

Other less frequent viral causes of oral lesions include cytomegalovirus ulcers, human papillomavirus. **Cytomegalovirus (CMV)** is a very common virus that most people have been exposed to long before they were exposed to HIV-1. Once the immune system malfunctions, the virus causes infection in the eyes, intestinal tract, and less commonly, the mucosal tissue. CMV is most often associated with retinitis, and mucosal involvement is uncommon. Oral ulcers are usually seen in the presence of disseminated disease. CMV ulcers can occur on any oral mucosal surface, and severe oral disease generally occurs in the context of systemic CMV infection. Intraoral CMV may present as nonspecific mucositis, large shallow ulcerations, or salivary gland enlargement and xerostomia (dry mouth). CMV has also been implicated as a cause of significant pharyngeal pain causing swallowing difficulties (Dichtel, 1992). Diagnosis of oral or oropharyngeal CMV disease is made by biopsy. Medical treatment consists of systemic antiviral drugs (Battinelli & Peters, 1993).

Human papillomavirus is the agent responsible for skin and mucosal warts. Human papillomavirus-associated warts have been noted with increased frequency in patients with AIDS than in the population at-large. Greenspan and associates (1990) have done extensive studies on human papillomavirus strains found in the oral cavities of HIV-1-infected persons and noted unusual strains to be present in increased frequencies in this population. The lesions were described as falling into three distinct categories of appearance: cauliflower, spiky, and flat. The warts may be removed surgically if warranted because of pain or interference with chewing, speaking, or swallowing. Recurrences of the warts are frequent even after surgical removal.

Neoplastic Diseases

The presence of **Kaposi's sarcoma** in an individual under the age of 60 meets the Centers for Disease Control and Prevention criteria for the definition of AIDS. Kaposi's sarcoma is second only to *Pneumocystis carinii* pneumonia as the most frequent AIDS manifestation. Kaposi's sarcoma is the most common neoplasm associated with AIDS, and more than 50% of patients with Kaposi's sarcoma have lesions in the mouth (Dodd, Greenspan & Greenspan, 1991; Schiodt & Pindborg, 1987).

Symptoms of Kaposi's sarcoma are raised or thickened tissue that is reddish or purplish in color. In early stages, the nodules may be the same color as the adjoining normal tissue. The tumors can cover a relatively small area in the mouth or they can cover the entire palate or gingival margin. The lesions of Kaposi's sarcoma may occur on any mucosal surface within the oral cavity but 95% are found on the palatal surfaces, especially the hard palate (Dichtel, 1992; Greenspan et al., 1990).

In many cases, the lesions may be painless and the tumors grow very slowly. Common complications of Kaposi's sarcoma in the mouth include pain, bleeding, and intrusion of the tumors onto the teeth causing tooth loss (Bartlett & Finkbeiner, 1993). Bulky lesions may be visible and may interfere with speech and mastication (Greenspan & Greenspan, 1995). In patients with AIDS, ulceration and bleeding occur in approximately 28% and dysphagia has been reported in 25% of the patients with oral Kaposi's sarcoma (Dichtel, 1992). Lesions on the gingival margin frequently become inflamed and painful because of plaque accumulation.

In the absence of pain, bleeding, or intrusion onto the teeth, the tumors are left untreated. When treatment is warranted, the tumors may be surgically removed or treated with radiation, lasers, or chemotherapy using cancer drugs (Bartlett & Finkbeiner, 1993; Phelan, 1997). Lesions may recur following treatment.

Another neoplastic disease associated with HIV-1 infection is **non-Hodgkin's lymphoma.** Although not seen as frequently as with oral Kaposi's sarcoma, oral lesions from non-Hodgkin's lymphoma are a common feature of HIV-1 infection. A biopsy may prove that nonspecific alveolar swellings or discrete oral masses on the palate or gingiva are non-Hodgkin's lymphoma. When occurring in the oral cavity, the lymphomas have appeared as necrotic, ulcerated, or nonulcerated masses (Phelan, 1997). When not ulcerated, the mass may be of normal color or look reddish and inflamed. Once the diagnosis is made with biopsy, current treatment is chemotherapy. The prognosis is generally poor (Dichtel, 1992; Phelan, 1997).

An HIV-related cancer that is found primarily on the tongue is **squamous cell carcinoma.** Lesions are usually found on the lateral and undersurface of the tongue (Battinelli & Peters, 1993). Treatment consists of surgical removal of the mass or radiation therapy. Resection and neck dissection may be indicated in some cases (Dichtel, 1992).

Other Oral Conditions

Recurrent aphthous ulcers, commonly called canker sores, are a common finding in the uninfected population. These lesions occur with greater frequency and greater severity in the HIV positive population (Dichtel, 1992; Phelan, 1997). Three forms of aphthous ulcerations have been described: minor, major, and herpetiform. **Minor aphthous ulcerations** occur on nonkeratinized oral mucosa. Therefore, minor aphthous ulcerations do not involve the hard palate, gingiva, or dorsum of the tongue because they are keratinized. Lesions appear as small, painful, shallow, round-to-oval ulcers on an inflamed base with a raised white, glistening margin. The small lesions will often coalesce into larger lesions (Dichtel, 1992). **Major aphthous ulcers** are larger than 1 cm in diameter and are deeper and last longer than minor ulcers. They are painful and often are located in the posterior part of the mouth. Lesions may be persistent and difficult to treat. **Herpetiform aphthous ulcers** are the rarest form of aphthous ulcers. Lesions are large, very painful, and may appear anywhere on the oral mucosa. Recurrent aphthous ulcers can interfere significantly with speech and swallowing (Greenspan & Greenspan, 1995).

Idiopathic thrombocytopenic purpura may produce small blood-filled lesions that contribute to spontaneous gingival bleeding (Battinelli & Peters, 1993; Dichtel, 1992; Greenspan & Greenspan, 1995). These lesions may be mistaken for Kaposi's sarcoma.

Salivary gland disease has been reported in HIV-1 seropositive adults. The patient may complain of dry mouth (xerostomia), and there may be signs of mucosal dryness, lack of pooled saliva, and failure to elicit salivary flow or reduced salivary production. **Xerostomia** has been reported to occur in 6 to 10% in persons with HIV-1 infection (Dichtel, 1992). The cause of the dry mouth is unknown but it may be related to CMV, side effects of medication, or salivary gland enlargement related to HIV-1 infection. Rinsing with saline solution and the use of sugarless gum may be helpful. The decrease in salivary flow increases the risk of cavities and inflammatory periodontal disease (Phelan, 1997). An additional discomfort associated with dry mouth is difficulty swallowing due to lack of saliva.

Diseases of the Nose and Paranasal Sinuses

Diseases of the nose and paranasal sinuses will affect resonance, causing the individual to sound chronically hyponasal. Bacterial sinusitis is a common complication of advanced HIV-1 infection and can be difficult to treat medically. Although the percentage of patients with symptoms specifically localized to the nose and paranasal sinuses is not precisely known, prospective studies of patients infected with HIV-1 have reported a 30 to 68% prevalence of sinusitis (Thompson, Salvato, Stroud, & Hasheeve, 1993; Zurlo, Feuerstein, Lebovics, & Lane, 1992). Patients with CD4 counts below 200 are particularly prone to develop chronic sinusitis involving multiple sinuses (Jacobson, 1995). Other sinonasal conditions that occur in people with HIV-1 infection and may affect resonance include adenoidal hypertrophy, allergy and allergic rhinitis, neoplasms, and inflammatory sinusitis.

Adenoidal hypertrophy is common during the course of HIV-1 infection. These patients present with lymphadenopathy (disease of the lymph tissue) and generalized proliferation of lymphoid tissue that includes adenoids and lingual and faucial tonsils (Tami & Wawrose, 1992). This correlation is so significant in the HIV-1-infected population that the occurrence of adenoidal hypertrophy in a nonpediatric patient, even if asymptomatic, should always raise the possibility of an underlying HIV-1 infection. Nasal obstruction is the most common complaint, and otitis media with effusion is a frequent associated finding (Tami & Wawrose, 1992).

Tami and Wawrose (1992) reported that in people with HIV-1 infection, there is a twofold increase in the incidence of **allergic rhinitis** (inflammation of the nasal mucosa) and associated allergic symptoms. There was a reported 41% incidence before infection and 87% after. Currently, it is unknown why this population has an increased incidence of allergic symptoms, although a defect of immune regulation is thought to be involved.

Malignant neoplasms (recent tumor or growth) that affect the sinonasal area include Kaposi's sarcoma, non-Hodgkin's lymphoma, and β cell lymphoma (Tami & Wawrose, 1992). Sinus, intranasal, and nasopharynx lesions are more uncommon than in other regions of the head and neck, such as the oral cavity and oropharynx. Presenting symptoms include nasal obstruction, intermittent nosebleeds, and runny nose.

Prospective studies have placed the prevalence of **inflammatory sinusitis** (inflammation of the paranasal mucosa) in the HIV-1-infected population at 20 to 68% (Rubin & Honigsberg, 1990). Diagnosis and treatment of acute sinusitis in this population are similar to that for non-HIV-1-infected persons. Presenting signs and symptoms include fever, headaches, stuffiness, and thick mucopurulent postnasal drainage from the infected sinus (Tami & Wawrose, 1992).

Ophthalmic Complications

Ophthalmic complications associated with HIV-1 are described in this section on head and neck manifestations because it is probable that visual deficits will be noted first during an initial evaluation of the patient when doing the oral-peripheral examination. Visual deficits, depending upon severity, negatively affect a person's reading, writing, and daily living activities and may compromise safety if living independently. It has been reported that more than 50% of patients with AIDS have ophthalmic changes associated with HIV-1 infection (Tay-Kearney & Jabs, 1996). Microvascular abnormalities and opportunistic infections cause the majority of ophthalmic lesions in this population.

The advent of more effective treatments of opportunistic infections has led to increased survival for patients with AIDS. This increased survival, in turn, has resulted in a rise in the frequency of cytomegalovirus (CMV) disease. **CMV retinitis** is the most common CMV disease reported. CMV retinitis generally occurs in the late stages of HIV-1 disease. Symptoms of CMV retinitis include deteriorating vision, seeing moving spots of different shapes and sizes (floaters), flashing lights (photopsias), and patches of blind spots (scotomata) (Tay-Kearney & Jabs, 1996). CMV retinitis can occur in one or both eyes. The severity of vision loss is determined by the site of lesion on the retina. If infection occurs in one eye and is untreated, it often will affect the other eye as well (Bartlett & Finkbeiner,

1993). If both eyes are infected and left untreated, the usual result is blindness.

If the lesion is small or peripheral, the patient may be asymptomatic. Patients becoming symptomatic will report painless visual loss that may range from blurred vision to loss of a portion of the visual field, and unilateral or bilateral flashes of light or floaters, eye redness, or pain (Jones & Molaghan, 1995). Floaters are spots that float across the line of vision as a result of inflamed cells in the middle of the eye. In HIV-1-related retinopathy (any disorder of the retina), subtle changes in color vision and contrast sensitivity have also been reported (Tay-Kearney & Jabs, 1996).

OTOLOGIC MANIFESTATIONS

Otologic and neurotologic manifestations associated with HIV-1 infection have been reported but they occur less frequently than head and neck manifestations. Most otologic infections associated with AIDS are caused by routine organisms and respond to standard therapy (Lalwani & Sooy, 1992). Complications of the external, middle, and inner ear have been reported, as well as CNS lesions that affect hearing ability. Otologic manifestations include Kaposi's sarcoma of the ear, *Pneumocystis carinii* otitis, eustachian tube obstruction secondary to nasopharyngeal mass, serous otitis media, auditory brain stem response abnormalities, and sensorineural hearing loss secondary to CNS complications of AIDS. Table 5–2 presents a summary of common otologic findings.

Outer and Middle Ear Manifestations

There are two outer ear manifestations of HIV-1 infection that may result in conductive hearing loss: otitis externa and Kaposi's sarcoma. Bacterial external otitis does occur in HIV-1 infection but the incidence is not significantly higher in persons with HIV-1 infection than in the general population (Marcusen & Sooy, 1985; Sooy, 1987). **Otitis externa** is an infection of the cartilaginous external canal and is typically associated with excessive irritation or mechanical trauma. Symptoms include ear canal inflammation with purulent debris obscuring the tympanic membrane. Depending on the severity of infection, stenosis of the ear canal may occur due to edema, causing a conductive hearing loss. Otitis externa in a person with HIV-1 responds well to standard antibiotic therapy (Morris & Prasad, 1990). In the immunosupressed population, external otitis may evolve into malignant otitis externa or osteomyelitis of the skull base (Lalwani & Sooy, 1992).

Table 5–2. Otologic manifestations associated with HIV-1 infection.

External Ear	Middle Ear	Inner Ear	CNS
otitis externa	serous otitis media	sensorineural hearing loss	central hearing loss
malignant otitis externa	eustachian tube dysfunction	iatrogenic hearing loss	mental status change
Kaposi's sarcoma	nasopharyngeal masses	ABR abnormality	necrosis of CN VIII
non-Hodgkin's lymphoma	acute otitis media	vertigo	endolymphatic hydrops
	mastoiditis		facial palsy

Another manifestation of HIV-1 infection that affects the external ear and may cause conductive hearing loss is Kaposi's sarcoma. Kaposi's sarcoma of the auricle is seen almost exclusively in individuals with AIDS (Marcusen & Sooy, 1985; Sooy, 1987). The sarcoma also may involve the external auditory canal, the tympanic membrane, and the middle ear, resulting in conductive hearing loss.

In addition to Kaposi's sarcoma, serous otitis media (SOM), large nasopharyngeal masses, acute otitis media (AOM), *Pneumocystis carinii* otitis media (PcOM), and mastoiditis have been reported to affect the middle ear in people infected with HIV-1 (Kohan, Hammerschlag, & Holiday, 1990; Lalwani & Sooy, 1992). The HIV-1-infected population is at greater risk of recurrent viral opportunistic infections, adenoidal hypertrophy, nasopharyngeal masses, or viral-induced allergies (see discussion of head and neck manifestations), which consequently may result in poor eustachian tube function (Lalwani & Sooy, 1992). Secondary to eustachian tube dysfunction, SOM, which is the presence of middle ear effusion without inflammation, may be more common in adults with AIDS (Marcusen & Sooy, 1985; Sooy, 1987).

Lawani and Sooy (1992) reported findings of nasal obstruction, otitis media with effusion, and conductive hearing loss in adult patients with HIV-1 infection. Another frequent finding was that of large benign nasopharyngeal masses due to proliferation of lymphoid tissue including adenoids and lingual and faucial tonsils. The occurrence of adenoidal hypertrophy in a nonpediatric patient, even if asymptomatic, should always raise the possibility of an underlying HIV-1 infection (Tami & Wawrose, 1992).

The bacterial causes and clinical manifestations of AOM in the HIV-1-positive population are similar to those of the noninfected population

(Lalwani & Sooy, 1992). However, *Pneumocystis carinii* **otitis media (PcOM)** is an opportunistic otologic infection unique to HIV-1 disease (Gherman, Ward, & Bassis, 1988; Kohan et al., 1990). Bacterial pneumococcal infection affects extrapulmonary sites by invasion of the bloodstream and, consequently, organs of the sinopulmonary system may be infected concomitantly and acutely by pneumococci (Duma, 1992). Infected organ structures include the sinuses (sinusitis), mastoids (mastoiditis), and ears (otitis media). Pneumococcal infection may enter the middle ear via the eustachian tube from a colonized nasopharynx. In addition, if the tympanic membrane is perforated, otitis externa may develop. Patients complain of otalgia (pain in the ear), otorrhea (discharge from the ear), and hearing loss with PcOM. Audiometric examination demonstrates a conductive or mixed hearing loss (Lalwani & Sooy, 1992).

Mastoiditis has been reported by several authors (Duma, 1992; Gherman et al., 1988; Kohan et al., 1990). Although chronic otitis media, cholesteatoma (a cyst-like sac filled with keratin debris that may grow to occlude the middle ear), intracranial complications of otitis media and other suppurative (pus producing) complications of ear infections are described in people who are HIV-1 positive, there is no evidence to suggest that these infections occur more frequently in these individuals.

Any of the external or middle ear manifestations can present with a mild to moderate conductive hearing loss characterized by the classic air-bone gap. Expected immitance findings are low-mobility tympanograms, negative pressure in the middle ear, and absence of acoustic reflexes (Madriz & Herrera, 1995). Because the opportunistic infections that affect the external and middle ear respond well to standard treatment, the associated hearing losses generally are reversible (Morris & Prasad, 1990; Lalwani & Sooy, 1992).

Inner Ear and Neurotologic Manifestations

Sensorineural hearing loss reported in persons with HIV-1 infection ranges from 20.9 to 49% (Lalwani & Sooy, 1992). The early CNS involvement and changing pattern of opportunistic infection has been shown to compromise the auditory nerve (Ollo et al., 1991). There is growing evidence of both central and peripheral hearing loss associated with opportunistic infections such as primary CNS lymphomas (Dichtel, 1992; Flower & Sooy, 1987; Lalwani & Sooy, 1992), herpes simplex and herpes zoster viruses (Wilson, 1986), cryptococcal and aseptic meningitis (Lewis & Rabinovich, 1972), and neurosyphilis (Gordon et al., 1994). The reader is referred to Chapter 4 for information on each of these CNS pathologies.

Sooy (1987) did a prospective study with audiograms of 53 patients diagnosed with AIDS at San Francisco General Hospital. Results revealed that 45% had sensorineural hearing loss defined as a hearing threshold worse than 25 dBHL. The typical audiogram demonstrated a sloping high-frequency loss. Two thirds of the patients had a loss between 30 and 50 dB HL at 8000Hz. Moderate to severe loss at three or more test frequencies (250 to 8000 Hz), in at least one ear, was present in one third of the patients. In the presence of these losses, the speech discrimination score was greater than 90% in the majority of patients and none of the scores were less than 82%.

Another study at San Francisco General Hospital studied auditory brainstem responses (ABRs) prospectively in 25 patients with confirmed diagnosis of AIDS and age- and sex-matched control subjects (Lalwani & Sooy, 1992). Study findings revealed that the ABR waveforms of the subjects with AIDS were highly degraded. AIDS was associated with normal Wave I latency and significantly prolonged Wave V latency. The interpeak latencies were prolonged in the HIV-1-infected group. The study concluded that the findings were similar to ABR results seen in demyelinating disease, and this result may be due to myelopathy that has been described in AIDS by Petito et al. (1985). Welkoborsky and Lowitzsch (1992) also reported that absolute and interwave ABR latencies were prolonged in individuals with AIDS.

The exact cause and site of lesion for sensorineural hearing loss associated with HIV-1 disease is unknown. Sensorineural hearing loss may involve a cochlear lesion, central lesion, or both. Lawani and Sooy (1992) concluded that prolonged absolute wave latencies may be associated with peripheral loss, but delayed neural conduction velocities suggest a retrocochlear lesion, and that ABR findings in AIDS patients support central auditory dysfunction, which partially explains the hearing loss.

Sensorineural hearing loss associated with HIV-1 may be caused by secondary opportunistic infections of the CNS or as a result of primary HIV-1 infection of the CNS. Many of the drugs used to treat HIV-1 infection and its complications are ototoxic, causing hearing loss. Another form of therapy that may cause sensorineural hearing loss is the use of radiation to treat CNS lymphomas associated with HIV-1.

The evaluation of hearing loss in the patient with AIDS should be approached as an VIIIth nerve cranial neuropathy (Lawani & Sooy, 1992). A complete audiogram with pure tone thresholds, speech audiometry, impedance audiometry, and acoustic reflexes should be performed. An ABR needs to be obtained to evaluate retrocochlear pathology. Aural rehabilitation with hearing aids and assistive listening devices should be instituted when there is significant hearing loss or auditory disability.

DYSPHAGIA

The digestive system includes the mouth, throat, esophagus, stomach, small intestine, large intestine or colon, and the anus. This system is responsible for oral intake of solids and liquids, digestion of the food, and elimination of waste. HIV-1 infection can affect any part of the digestive system and commonly does so during the late stages of the disease (Tanowitz et al., 1996; Wilcox, 1992; Wilcox et al., 1993). The symptoms or patient complaints indicate which part of the digestive system is being affected.

Painful or difficult chewing indicates a problem in the mouth. Pain upon swallowing or difficulty swallowing indicate problems in the pharynx or esophagus. Pain in the chest after swallowing is due to an esophageal problem. Abdominal pain, nausea, and vomiting generally are due to stomach complications. Diarrhea, cramping, and malnutrition from the failure to absorb nutrients are all symptoms of problems with the small intestine. Pain, chronic diarrhea, and constipation are symptoms of problems with the colon.

Primary HIV-1 infection is responsible for substantial weight loss. The frequency and importance of weight loss in AIDS resulted in the 1987 inclusion of the **HIV wasting syndrome** in the revised Centers for Disease Control surveillance case definition. Weight loss of greater than 10% occurs in 62 to 79% of persons as a result of primary HIV-1 infection (Kotler, Wang, & Pierson, 1985; O'Sullivan, Linke, & Dalton, 1985). Causes of weight loss and malnutrition in HIV-1 disease are multifactorial (Heffernan, Osten, & Dunn, 1993). The problems of the digestive system place the individual with HIV-1 infection at an increased risk for weight loss and malnutrition.

It was noted as early as 1981 that difficulty swallowing **(dysphagia)** and pain on swallowing **(odynophagia)** were common complaints in HIV-infected patients, particularly among those with advanced stage of infection. In one study of 71 adult males with HIV-1 infection, dysphagia was noted in 21% of the cases (Chelbowski et al., 1989). Odynophagia, which is usually due to esophageal involvement, is described in up to 90% of patients with AIDS (Afdhal, 1995).

Esophageal Diseases

Esophageal diseases are associated with dysphagia, odynophagia, and chest pain in individuals with HIV-1 infection (Friedman, 1994; Rabeneck et al., 1990). Pain on swallowing frequently is an indication of the presence of invasive infection of the esophagus. Esophageal candidiasis is the most frequent cause of dysphagia and odynophagia in patients with HIV-1 infection and accounts for 48 to 75% of esophageal symptoms in AIDS patients (Raufman, 1988; Wilcox, Zaki, & Coffield, 1993). However, not all patients with esophageal disease exhibit symptoms of dysphagia, odynophagia, or both.

When inflammation of the esophagus occurs, it is termed **esophagitis.** Esophagitis, occurring in the absence of any known predisposing condition, is an indication of HIV-1 infection. Infection with *Candida albicans* is the most common cause of symptomatic esophageal complaints in AIDS. *Candida albicans* is part of the normal flora of the body but also may be recovered from the soil, hospital environments, food, and other substrates.

Candida may occur alone or in association with other infectious pathogens, including cytomegalovirus (CMV), herpes simplex virus (HSV) or, in rare cases, opportunistic infections such as *Mycobacterium tuberculosis* or *Cryptosporidium* organisms (Friedman, 1994). CMV and idiopathic ulcers are more likely to produce odynophagia and esophagospasm than dysphagia (Wilcox, 1993). Rabeneck and associates (1990) reported that acute HIV infection may be associated with esophageal ulcers that result in odynophagia, dysphagia, and **esophagospasm** (spasm of the esophagus).

Some gastrointestinal manifestations are the result of the drugs used to prolong life in the fight against AIDS. The widespread use of prophylaxis for opportunistic pathogens, while promoting longer survival for AIDS patients, also may increase gastrointestinal diseases (Tanowitz et al, 1996). Two drugs that have been reported to cause drug-related esophagitis are zidovudine (ZDV) and dideoxycytidine (ddC).

Esophageal obstruction may be caused by primary non-Hodgkin's lymphoma (NHL) and Kaposi's sarcoma. Gastrointestinal tract involvement of HIV-1-related lymphoma is found in 10 to 25% of patients with AIDS (Straus, 1997). There is indication that the incidence of NHL is increasing in the HIV-infected population. Improved medical management of opportunistic infections and advances in antiretroviral treatment have combined to increase the life span of an HIV-infected persons but these people remain in an immunosuppressed state. There is increased risk of developing unusual types of NHL due to this weakened immune state.

The current medical treatment of esophageal symptoms in AIDS includes a variety of antifungal agents. Because *Candida* is the most common cause of esophagitis, the use of drug therapy for one week to determine if symptoms were alleviated was found to be more cost-effective than initial endoscopy (Wilcox et al., 1993). If there is no improvement with drugs within seven days, endoscopy is performed. The diagnosis of esophageal ulcers from CMV, HSV, and other pathogens is confirmed by biopsy of tissue obtained endoscopically from the center of the ulcer. Most patients with *Candida* esophagitis relapse (Tanowitz et al., 1996) and esophageal lesions may persist despite prolonged therapy. It is not unusual for esophagitis to recur once drugs are discontinued.

Medical treatment for esophageal obstruction secondary to primary lymphomas and Kaposi's sarcoma generally involves chemotherapy. The majority of patients with HIV-associated non-Hodgkin's lymphoma (NHL) do not respond well with conventional chemotherapy. A number of investigators are currently studying therapeutic methods that combine modified doses of chemotherapy with prophylactic intervention.

The specific cause of swallowing dysfunction in an individual with HIV-1 infection is very complex to identify. The presence of multiple concomitant infecting organisms makes it difficult to ascribe a symptom or sign to a single pathogen.

Oropharyngeal Lesions

The oral and pharyngeal lesions associated with HIV-1-related opportunistic infections was discussed at length earlier in this chapter. Table 5–1 presented a summary of the fungal, bacterial, viral, neoplastic, and miscellaneous conditions that may result in oral manifestations related to HIV-1 disease. Lesions on the gingiva, tongue, palate, and buccal mucosa contribute to dysphagia by impeding mastication and oral management of bolus. Oropharyngeal lesions may cause pain and dysphagia during the pharyngeal phase of swallow.

Issues in Nutritional Support

Swallowing difficulties interfere with nutrition. Anything that interferes with nutrition is especially important to an individual with HIV-1 infection because the virus itself causes weight loss and nutritional deficiencies. Severe malnutrition also seems to weaken the immune system further. Therefore, the primary goals of nutritional support are preservation of lean body mass and provision of adequate protein, calories, and other essential nutrients in a diet that minimizes side effects, especially malabsorption. Currently, there is no clinically proven superior oral, enteral (such as nasogastric or gastronomy tube), or parenteral (intravenous feeding) diet for patients with symptomatic HIV-1 disease (Heffernan et al., 1993).

Nutritional support is indicated if a patient has lost 20 pounds or 10% of body weight in 6 months or is unable to meet 100% of his or her nutritional needs (Hickey & Weaver, 1988). Maintaining safe oral intake of nutrients is preferable because it maintains structural and functional integrity of the gastrointestinal mucosa, minimizes cost, and decreases risk of infection. The patient may require enteral feeding via a nasogastric tube to supplement oral intake due to dysphagia or odynophagia. If oral intake of nutrition is inadequate for more than three consecutive days for patients who are sick enough to be hospitalized, tube feedings should be considered (Heffernan et al., 1993). With long-term dysfunction of the esophagus or upper digestive tract, placement of a gastronomy or jejunostomy (surgical opening into the second portion of the small intestines) tube is recommended (Heffernan et al., 1993). When esophageal ulcers preclude the use of nasogastric tube feedings, short term (7–10 days) parenteral nutrition may be considered.

A severely malnourished person may need parenteral nutrition via intravenous feeding to reestablish nutritional homeostasis. In this mode, nutrients are delivered directly to the cells by infusion into the bloodstream rather than by way of digestive system. This type of feeding may be required if severe malabsorption of nutrients occurs in the digestive system or if rapid correction of nutritional deficiencies is needed to prepare a patient for impending surgery. However, this method of providing nutrition is expensive and not recommended routinely. The decision to implement chronic parenteral nutritional support should be made only after careful assessment of its likely effect on quality and duration of life. A patient receiving total parenteral nutrition should be reevaluated every four to six weeks to assess the degree of success of parenteral feeding and its affect on the patient's quality of life.

A low-fat, soft, bland diet with dietary supplements is recommended for patients who safely tolerate an oral diet. However, if eating is painful, patients tend to lose their appetite. Such patients should avoid spices and acids that will cause pain to ulcerations. They should try soft consistencies that will not irritate the mouth or throat. In patients with disorders of the oral cavity, pharynx, and esophagus, modifications in the acidity, temperature, texture, consistency, and seasoning of food may improve tolerance. Patients should be provided instruction in basic safe swallow strategies, such as eating in an upright position, taking small bites of food, thorough chewing, refraining from talking while chewing and swallowing, and eating at a moderate pace.

If eating is no longer pleasurable due to psychological or emotional issues, it may be helpful to implement relaxation exercises before meals and to offer small frequent feedings during the course of the day. Efforts to make eating a special event may be beneficial, such as use of pleasant music, fixing food to look attractive, eating with a friend, and preparing favorite foods. In addition to frequent, small meals, nutritious and high-calorie snacks should be readily available.

CHAPTER SUMMARY

HIV-1-related complication in the head and neck region are very common. Nearly 100% of persons with AIDS report head and neck manifestations during the course of the disease. These include oropharyngeal lesions, nasopharyngeal lesions, ophthalmic complications, and otologic manifestations. HIV-1-related opportunistic infections that cause these varied pathologies are treated in a variety of ways medically.

Persons with late stage HIV-1 infection and AIDS commonly report dysphagia or odynophagia. Lesions of mouth and esophagus are frequent because these areas are particularly vulnerable to infection in persons with weakened immune systems. The orpharynx and digestive tract naturally host a multitude of microflora. When the immune system becomes weakened, the microflora grow unchecked, creating lesions that interfere with chewing, swallowing, and digestion. This condition further complicates metabolic imbalances that are the result of HIV-1 in the body.

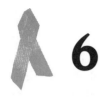 **6**

Pediatric HIV-1 Infection

Since the first reported case in 1982 (CDC, 1982e), pediatric AIDS has emerged as a major public health problem. The impact of the pediatric HIV-1 epidemic is unique among illnesses that have confronted society in modern times. The disease often affects multiple members of a single household. At the current rate of transmission, the number of orphans under 10 years of age worldwide may approach 10 million by the end of the century (Chin, 1994; Wiznia, Lambert, & Pavlakis, 1996).

During the early history of HIV-1, most of the children who were identified died within a short period of time, tragically minimizing concerns about neuropsychological or developmental deficits. However, early identification of children at risk for HIV-1 infection combined with advances in medical management now extend life expectancy for children with HIV-1 and AIDS. With extended life expectancy, issues including speech and language development, learning disabilities, hearing deficits, and special educational needs will need to be addressed. Communication disorders specialists and special education professionals must acquire adequate information about HIV-1 and its effect on infected children. This chapter will present information on pediatric AIDS, its epidemiology and transmission, natural history, clinical manifestations of infection, and associated neuropsychological, developmental, and educational deficits.

EPIDEMIOLOGY AND TRANSMISSION

In the United States, from 1979 to 1982, children were identified who had illnesses suggestive of AIDS; however, the first case was not reported until 1982 (CDC, 1982e). The incidence of AIDS in the pediatric population has risen significantly as the disease has spread in the United States. Approximately 7,000 infants are born annually to women with HIV-1 infection (CDC, 1994b). The number of HIV-1-infected children in the United States is estimated at 10,000 to 20,000, with approximately 80% under the age of 5 years (Jenkins, 1996).

HIV-1 infection was first identified mainly in children exposed to the virus through transfusion of HIV-1-infected blood or blood products due to coagulant disorders, chronic anemia, or hematologic disorders requiring multiple transfusions. Although there were early reports of HIV-1 infection in infants born to intravenous drug users or to women who had multiple sexual partners (Novick, 1989), the majority of pediatric infections were due to receiving infected blood. The virus entered the U. S. blood supply in the mid to late 1970s, and by 1981–1982, more than 50% of patients with severe hemophilia had become infected with HIV-1 (Eyster et al., 1985). Since 1985, the screening of blood products has virtually eliminated new infections from transfusions (Jenkins, 1996; Pizzo, 1990).

Since 1985, the fastest growing group of children with HIV-1 infection and related disorders are infants who are infected through perinatal transmission (Minkoff, Nanda, Menez, & Fikrig, 1987; Wolinsky et al., 1992). Perinatal or vertical transmission (occurring from infected mother to infant before, during, or shortly after birth) accounts for nearly 90 to 95% of AIDS cases in children younger than 13 (CDC, 1994b; Jenkins, 1996; Wara & Dorenbaum, 1995).

Estimates of rates of transmission of HIV-1 from infected mother to infant ranges from 13 to 40% (Griffith & Booss, 1994). Perinatal transmission of the virus can occur during pregnancy (in utero or prenatal period), during the actual birth process (intrapartum), and during the first month of life (neonatal period). During the neonatal period, transmission through breast-feeding has been described (Goldfarb, 1993).

In the United States, the disease disproportionately affects African-American and Hispanic women and children (CDC, 1994c). AIDS rate for African-American women is 16 times higher than those for white women. The rate is 7 times higher for Hispanic women than for white women. Various high-risk activities are reported among women with HIV-1 infection: 41% reported intravenous drug use; 38% reported heterosexual contact with a partner who engaged in at-risk behavior or was known to be HIV-1-positive; 2% reported contaminated blood products; and 19% had no reported risk factor. Children account for approximately 2% of AIDS cases in the United States.

The incidence of HIV-1 infection associated with heterosexual contact has continued to increase, primarily reflecting transmission from the large population of intravenous drug users to their heterosexual partners (CDC, 1997). In 1997, the largest increase of infection was in women within the age range of 25–44. Because these women are of childbearing age, there will be parallel growth in incidence of perinatally transmitted HIV-1 infection (Anastos, Denenberg, & Solomon, 1997; Belman, 1992).

In February 1994, a randomized, placebo-controlled study (Connors et al., 1994) demonstrated that the use of zidovudine (AZT) effected a remarkable 67.5% reduction in mother-to-child transmission of HIV-1 compared to the placebo group. The women studied had not previously received long-term zidovudine therapy and were in the early stages of HIV-1 disease.

In the study (Connors et al., 1994), zidovudine was administered to HIV-1-infected pregnant women during late pregnancy and intrapartum and to their infants in the early neonatal period. The study group experienced 8.3% perinatal transmission versus 25.5% perinatal transmission in the placebo group. Study results revealed that the reduction in perinatal transmission was due solely to the zidovudine therapy. The researchers concluded that zidovudine therapy did reduce perinatal transmission of HIV-1 by two thirds but it did not completely eliminate the risk because some of the study group infants did acquire HIV-1 infection despite zidovudine treatment. The result of AIDS clinical trial group (ACTG) protocol 076 became highly publicized, capturing the attention of the scientific world as well as the popular media.

As discussed above, infants and young children are most frequently infected with HIV-1 through perinatal transmission. Adolescents (ages 13–18), however, are infected primarily due to risky personal health choices. It is estimated that 25% of HIV-1 infections are contracted during adolescence (Solorio & Stevens, 1997). Examples of risky behavior include unprotected sex with multiple partners, intravenous drug use, and alcohol use that impairs judgment. Contracting HIV-1 infection is a particular risk to runaway teens who engage in prostitution to survive. A very small but notable group of HIV-positive children and adolescents are the victims of sexual abuse (Jenkins, 1996).

NATURAL HISTORY OF HIV-1 INFECTION

Perinatally infected infants do not show any clinical signs of infection at birth (Jenkins, 1996; Wiznia et al., 1996). These infants are clinically and immunologically normal but other complicating factors frequently are present. The developmental vulnerability of the central nervous system of a developing embryo and neonate may account for the relative frequency of encephalopathy reported in pediatric HIV-1 infection (Jenkins, 1996). A significant number of perinatally infected infants are affected by drug exposure in utero due to the high incidence of intravenous drug use by the mothers. In addition, exposure to HIV-1 antigens (a substance that induces the formation of antibodies to that substance) may place these infants at greater risk for developing chronic respiratory and pulmonary disease (Pizzo, 1990). The interval before symptoms occur is shorter in perinatally exposed children than in adults.

Perinatally infected infants have been divided into two groups according to the timing of vertical transmission (from mother to child): those infected in utero and those infected during the birth process (intrapartum) (Wiznia et al., 1996). Infants infected in utero comprise 30 to 50% of vertical transmissions and have detectable virus within 48 hours of birth; intrapartum exposure constitutes 50 to 70%, and these infants remain virus-negative until 7 to 90 days of life (Wara & Dorenbaum, 1995). Infants infected by breast-feeding were not grouped because this type of transmission occurs very rarely.

Preliminary information from studies suggests that those infected in utero tend to have high viral loads due to a rapid burst of viral replication shortly after birth resulting in a rapid decline of CD4+ lymphocytes. Infants exposed to HIV-1 in utero demonstrate more rapid disease progression when compared to infected infants with negative detectable virus in the first week of life (Grossman, 1995; Wiznia et al., 1996).

Children with HIV-1 infection are classified as rapid progressors or slow progressors. **Rapid progressors** are children who develop symptoms of HIV-1 infection during the first year of life and progress to AIDS by 5 years of age. Although the onset of symptoms is variable in the United States, the average age of onset of severe immunodeficiency ranges from 5 to 10 months, with 50 to 90% of infants becoming ill by their first birthday (Grossman, 1995).

Slow progressors remain asymptomatic for a longer period of time. In the first year of life, these children demonstrate a slower rate of CD4+ lymphocyte attrition, which suggests effective viral suppression by their immune systems. Few vertically infected infants remain asymptomatic beyond the third year of life (Grossman, 1995). However, there are reports of vertically infected long-term nonprogressors (Jansen, 1995).

A cross-sectional survey of 374 children older than 8 years of age revealed that 7% were asymptomatic, and an additional 11% had mild symptoms. Cases of spontaneous clearance of HIV-1 infection in perinatally infected children have also been reported (Bryson, 1995). Similar findings have been found in uninfected sexual partners of infected individuals and seronegative recipients of contaminated blood products. These groups of adults and children are being extensively studied.

CLINICAL MANIFESTATIONS
OF PEDIATRIC HIV-1 INFECTION

Although many HIV-1-related clinical manifestations in adults and children are the same, important differences do exist. As discussed in Chapter 2, the stages of HIV-1 infection in adults are acute infection phase, followed by seroconversion, and then an asymptomatic period during which the person feels well and functions normally. In approximately 5 to 8 years after seroconversion, the progression to early symptomatic infection occurs. Eight to 10 years after seroconversion, adults typically reach late symptomatic stage of infection, which is marked by severe opportunistic infections and the diagnosis of AIDS. Children with HIV-1 infection experience more rapid disease progression than infected adults.

The goal of this section is to provide a brief summary of information regarding HIV-1-related medical complications unique to children with the virus.

Opportunistic Infections

One of the major differences between pediatric and adult HIV-1 and AIDS is that opportunistic infections are more devastating to the adult population. Adults have been exposed throughout their lifetime to the variety of viral and bacterial agents that cause the opportunistic infections in them. When their immune system was intact, these infection-causing agents were dormant in the body. However, as the immune system becomes compromised, the infectious agents have opportunity to become active. Children, especially infants, have not been exposed to the majority of these infection-causing agents. Of the more than one dozen specific opportunistic infections that plague adults with HIV-1 infection, only three principal opportunistic infections in the pediatric population have been reported: *Pneumocystis carinii* pneumonia (Grossman, 1995; Jenkins, 1996), oral and esophageal candidiasis (Grossman, 1995; Jenkins, 1996; Phelan, 1997), and *Mycobacterium avium* complex (Jenkins, 1996; Wiznia et al., 1996).

Pneumocystis carinii pneumonia (PCP) is the most common opportunistic infection in pediatric HVI-1 infection. In infected children, PCP typically occurs during the first year of life. The median age for presentation is 9 months of age, although there is a peak at age 3 to 6 months among rapidly progressing infants (Jenkins, 1996).

Children with HIV-1 infection also develop opportunistic oropharyngeal lesions. Oral candidiasis and *candida* esophagitis are the most commonly reported. Just as in the adult population, these lesions may contribute to anorexia and dysphagia due to pain when eating or swallowing. Decreased oral intake may lead to malnutrition, contributing to metabolic imbalances and failure to thrive.

Mycobacterium avium complex, which is found in water, soil, and dairy products, rarely causes illness in the first year of life, but the likelihood of infection increases with the child's age. Symptoms of infection may include enlarged liver, inflammation of the lung, unexplained prolonged fever, weight loss, diarrhea, anemia, and muscle wasting.

Lymphoid Interstitial Pneumonitis

Lymphoid interstitial pneumonitis (LIP) is a chronic infiltration of the lungs and may severely limit the quality of a child's life due to progressive hypoxia (deficiency of oxygen) (Wiznia et al., 1996). LIP has been described in a small number of HIV-1-infected adults but has been reported more frequently in infected children. Various studies report a prevalence of LIP in approximately 20% (Jenkins, 1996) to 40% (Grossman, 1995) of the pediatric population with HIV-1 infection.

Bacterial Infections

Children with perinatally transmitted HIV-1 infection are more susceptible to bacterial infections than are infected adults (Kovacs, Leaf, & Simberkoff, 1997; Miller & Remington, 1991; Walsh & Butler, 1991). Exposure to the virus at a time when an infant's immune system is developing compromises an infant's defenses, resulting in impaired ability to mount effective antibody responses against infections. An infant also has had no prior exposure to bacterial infections; therefore, the immune system has not had an opportunity to develop specific antibodies to the bacteria. However, adults have a preexisting immune system with specific antibodies that provide some degree of protection against common bacterial pathogens. Bacterial pneumonias, otitis media, sinusitis, urinary tract infection, skin and soft tissue infection, meningitis, and other bacterial infections affect 15% (Jenkins, 1996) to 24% (Wiznia et al, 1996) of the pediatric HIV-1 population.

Failure to Thrive

Infants who are perinatally infected with HIV-1 fail to thrive (Scott et al., 1989). **Failure to thrive** means that the infant does not grow or develop according to normal or expected rate. This can include low birth weight, growth retardation, and poor cognitive development. It can also indicate a plateau in development or the loss of attained developmental milestones. Growth failure is a common and important finding in pediatric HIV-1 infection and is nearly always multifactorial (Jenkins, 1996; Wiznia et al., 1996).

HIV-1 can cause failure to grow in nonperinatally infected children, also. A study by Brettler, Forsberg, Bolivar, Brewster, and Sullivan (1990) revealed that children with hemophilia and asymptomatic HIV-1 infection showed growth retardation and that onset of growth failure was a reliable prognostic indicator for the progression of HIV-1 infection to AIDS. In some cases, the growth retardation occurred before any significant drop in CD4 cells could be measured. Thus, growth abnormalities in asymptomatic children should be considered an early sign of progression towards symptomatic disease.

Failure to thrive may be due to a variety of HIV-1-associated disorders including anorexia, hypermetabolism, central nervous system deficits, malabsorption of nutrients, and chronic or recurrent diarrhea. Poor nutritional intake may be due in part to pain related to oropharyngeal lesions (refer to Chapter 5 for a discussion of oropharyngeal manifestations related to HIV-1) and middle ear pathology, dysphagia secondary to neurologic dysfunction, or socioeconomic factors (such as a mother who is drug-dependent or poverty and resulting malnutrition).

Neurologic Disease

The incidence of central nervous system (CNS) disease in infants and children with HIV-1 infection is approximately 60% in children in advanced disease stage and 8% in asymptomatic children (Belman, 1992). The CNS disease syndrome associated with pediatric AIDS is HIV-associated encephalopathy. The most frequent manifestations are developmental delays, cognitive impairments, acquired microcephaly (reduced head size due to white matter abnormalities and calcification in the basal ganglia), bilateral corticospinal tract signs, and ataxia (Belman, 1990; Epstein et al., 1985; Kozlowski, 1992; Krasinski, Borkowsky, & Holzman, 1989). The severity of these symptoms varies and the rate of progression may be subacute progressive, plateau with either deterioration or improvement, or static.

Belman (1990, 1992) and Belman and associates (1985; Belman, Lantos et al., 1986; Belman, Ultmann et al., 1986) have extensively studied encephalopathy in pediatric HIV-1 infection. From their work, it is known that progressive encephalopathy has a profound effect on infants and young children. One may see deterioration of play, decreased vocalizations, or loss of previously acquired language and socialization skills. Progressive motor dysfunction is common and often results in loss of milestones. For example, the infant who was able to sit without support can no longer do so, or the infant who was pulling up to stand and beginning to take a few steps can no longer bear weight on his or her legs. The toddler who was walking independently has a change in gait, begins to walk on his her toes and, as the disease progresses, is unable to stand without assistance. These corticospinal tract signs are generally progressive and, with time, may result in spastic paraparesis (weakness of upper extremities) or quadriparesis (weakness of upper and lower extremities).

With progression of disease, most children become apathetic, lose interest in play and the environment, and exhibit decreased gestures and vocalizations. Chronic or recurrent otitis media is found in this population of children (Principi et al., 1991). Severely affected infants and young children may have a characteristic facial appearance. They appear alert but have an expressionless face and lack spontaneous facial expression and reduced eye blink. Microcephaly due to deceleration of head growth is common. If death from infection or cancer does not intervene, the child at the end-stage of disease is mute, dull-eyed, and quadriplegic. In some patients, deterioration is rapid and occurs in only 1 to 2 months. In others, the disease progression is episodic, with periods of deterioration interrupted by periods of relative neurologic stability.

The majority of children experience a plateau course of encephalopathy, which is a slower progression. Cognitive impairment is only evident as the rate of mental developmental progress declines. Although these children may continue to gain further cognitive, language, and socially adaptive skills, the rate of acquisition of these skills is slow. The rate of acquisition, relative to same-age peers, is below the norm and is also below their previous rate of developmental progress. These children function at a mental age lower than their chronologic age.

In plateau course, motor involvement is usually present, but progression and severity vary. Some children will develop corticospinal tract signs (e.g., gait disturbances, fine motor deficits, and inability to maintain standing balance or bear weight on legs) while others have less severe motor involvement that remains stable for long periods of time. Acquired microcephaly is evident but occurs much more slowly than in progressive encephalopathy. As the disease progresses, the plateau course may be followed by further deterioration that becomes similar to subacute progressive encephalopathy. For other children, the plateau may be followed by improvement. Over time, these children steadily gain additional developmental skills, and the rate of acquisition accelerates compared with their acquisition during plateau. Unfortunately, as continued follow-up over several years has documented, many of these children develop further neurologic problems related to HIV-1 CNS disease (Belman, 1990; Belman, Lantos, et al., 1986; Belman, Ultmann, et al., 1986).

Static, or stable, encephalopathy is characterized by continued but impaired development. The prevalence rate for static encephalopathy is estimated at 25%. In this group, the children acquire new skills and abilities at a rate consistent with their level of functioning during baseline testing. These children do have delays in acquisition of language and motor milestones but do not demonstrate loss of milestones.

Cerebrovascular Accidents

Cerebrovascular accidents (CVAs) occur in pediatric HIV-1 infection due to hemorrhage associated with thrombocytopenia. **Thrombocytopenia** is an abnormal deficiency of blood platelets. Platelets play an important role in blood coagulation, hemostasis (proper circulation of blood), and blood thrombus (clot) formation. The reported frequency of CVAs in the pediatric HIV-1 population is 1.3% (Belman, 1992; Wiznia et al., 1996). CVAs may be catastrophic and fatal or clinically insignificant in this population.

COMMUNICATION DISORDERS AND LEARNING DISABILITIES IN PEDIATRIC HIV-1

A large number of children with HIV-1 infection will exhibit a developmental disability or be at risk for one (Diamond, 1989; Diamond & Cohen, 1992; Kletter, Jeremy, Rumsey, Weintraub, & Cowan, 1989). Depending on the severity and progressive nature of CNS involvement, functional impairments of speech, language, cognition, hearing, and swallow will be evident (Belman, 1990). A well-controlled study of children hospitalized with AIDS revealed a high rate of cognitive delays (90%) and severe neurological involvement (100%) in the pediatric AIDS population (Diamond et al., 1990). Because there are communication disorders and dysphagia that are unique to this population, it is important that speech-language pathologists and audiologists become knowledgeable about treating children with HIV-1 infection.

Communication Disorders and Dysphagia

Pressman (1992), as part of the Children's Hospital AIDS Program (CHAP), provided speech-language pathology services from 1984 to 1992 to 150 children with AIDS. In an article published in *ASHA*, Pressman reviewed the conditions of 96 children seen in 1988 and 1989. The children were between the ages of 4 months and 17 years of age. Of the 96 subjects, 42 were boys and 54 were girls. Ninety-nine percent of the children were perinatally infected with HIV-1. The children were primarily from single parent families and were from low socioeconomic background. Baseline data gathered in the initial session were presented for these 96 children.

Children with HIV-1 infection demonstrate a large variety of communication disorders and dysphagia and the severity of deficits was in relation to disease progression (Pressman, 1992; Pressman & Morrison, 1988). Intervention for communication disorders related to static HIV-1 encephalopathy is the same as for any child with developmental delays, regardless of HIV status. However, children with progressive encephalopathy require a different intervention. Pressman (1992) did not elaborate on how this therapy would differ. An early sign of progressive encephalopathy is a decreased score on expressive vocabulary tests with concomitant increased gesturing and fillers in conversational speech. For children aged 3 years or older, vocabulary tests were found to be very sensitive to change in neurological status.

Decrease in mean length of utterance (MLU) was noted as another early sign of progressive encephalopathy. However, decreased MLU also may be secondary to chronic lung infections which plague the HIV-1-infected pediatric population. Lung infections contribute to respiratory insufficiency or breath support needed for speech. If the decreased MLU is due to respiratory insufficiency, MLU will improve as the lung infection is improved. If reduction of MLU is related to disease progression, improvement will not be seen, and verbal expression will be limited to occasional words and short phrases. Articulation becomes impaired and speech may be highly unintelligible due to the development of dysarthria. According to Pressman, this form of dysarthria does not show improvement through typical motor speech therapy.

As the encephalopathy progresses, deficits in receptive language will become evident. Receptive language remains more intact than expressive language skills. Therefore, the speech-language pathologist may recommend the use of sign language and augmentative means to enhance communication. Unfortunately, the motor impairments associated with progressive encephalopathy will cause the loss of fine motor movements needed to gesture, point, and use an augmentative communication device. When motor control is lost, patients and caretakers should be instructed in the use of eye gaze to communicate basic wants.

The following is a brief summary of the data presented in the study:

- 62 (69%) had deficits in **receptive language** that ranged from moderate to profound impairment. Some children with progressive encephalopathy were adequately tested for expressive language but could not be tested receptively due to severe motor impairments that inhibited a pointing response.
- 69 (75%) of the children had **expressive language** deficits.
- 3 (3%) had **sensorineural hearing loss** unrelated to AIDS and had previously been fitted with amplification.
- 3 (3%) suffered **CVAs.**
- 19 (19.8%) were **developmentally delayed** and had significant motor involvement and microcephaly.
- 6 (7.3%) had progressive encephalopathy including regression of motor skills, loss or regression in **expressive language,** and **dysarthria.**

- 26 (27%) had **articulation deficits.** The majority of these articulation deficits (65%) were mild to moderate in severity and consisted of developmental errors.
- 5 (19%) had poor **intelligibility** with a significant degree of assimilation and weak syllable deletion.
- 2 (7.6%) had **dysarthria** secondary to progressive encephalopathy.
- 2 (7.6%) had severe **motor speech disorders** secondary to CVA. The 2 children with severe dysarthria secondary to progressive encephalopathy and the 2 children with motor speech disorder secondary to CVA learned to use sign language, augmentative communication devices, or both.
- 12 (12.5%) had **voice disorders.** Of these, 2 (17%) had denasal and hoarse vocal quality, 8 (67%) had hoarse vocal quality, and 2 (17%) had weak and hypernasal vocal quality. Seven out of 8 of the hoarse voices were mild and 1 had a history of oral candidiasis. The 2 children with weak and hypernasal voices had progressive encephalopathy.
- 20 (20.8%) reported **dysphagia.** Complaints included coughing on food or liquids, slow feeding, failure to thrive, and gagging on solids or chewables. Of these children, oral preparatory, and oral and pharyngeal dysphagia problems were most common.
- Etiologies for dysphagia included static and progressive encephalopathy, neuromuscular discoordination, and oral and esophageal infections.
- Due to the significant psychosocial impact of HIV-1 infection, speech-language pathologists and audiologists must be aware of issues concerning mental health, cultural values, family and socioeconomic factors. The pediatric HIV-1 population may have communication disorders unrelated to their HIV status because they are born into high-risk families.

In addition to speech, language, and cognitive deficits, the pediatric population infected with HIV-1 may demonstrate recurrent otitis media due to their unique susceptibility to bacterial infections. Acute otitis media generally occurs due to bacterial infection of the respiratory tract by *Pneumocystis carinii* and *Candida* (Madriz & Herrera, 1995; Respler & Karas, 1996). Most cases of recurrent otitis media, if that is the only form of recurrent infection, are not due to HIV-1 infection but due to other factors that place the child at risk for middle ear pathology (e.g., eustachian tube dysfunction) (Bluestone & Klein, 1996). A few children will have recurrent otitis media as part of an immunodeficiency syndrome.

Otitis media may be more prevalent in children with HIV-1 infection and may be more difficult to eradicate than in children with intact immune systems (Haddad, Brager, & Bluestone, 1992). It has been found that eustachian tube dysfunction is more common in the pediatric AIDS population (Respler & Karas, 1996). This may be due to recurrent upper respiratory infections, adenoidal hypertrophy causing obstruction, or to HIV-1 infection itself.

In addition to middle ear pathology, sensorineural hearing loss has been reported in children with HIV-1 infection (Haddad et al., 1992; Madriz & Herrera, 1995; Pressman, 1992). Also, as a result of CNS damage due to HIV-1, central auditory processing disturbances have been reported (Belman, 1992; Madriz & Herrera, 1995). See Chapter 5 for a more in-depth discussion of audiologic involvement associated with HIV-1 infection.

Educational Challenges in Pediatric HIV-1

The effect of HIV-1 infection of the CNS presents a special challenge for educators and other professionals working with these children. The effect of the disease on each individual is different, causing global impairments in some children and specific deficits in others, and the rate of disease progression is unpredictable. This lack of predictability or uniformity makes early identification and intervention of HIV-1-related developmental abnormalities difficult.

Early signs of CNS impairment in school-aged children with HIV-1-associated progressive encephalopathy may include loss of interest in school performance and decline in academic progress (Belman, 1990; Belman et al., 1986; Brouwers, Belman, & Epstein, 1991). Additional signs include social withdrawal, increased emotional lability, attention deficits or worsening attention-deficit hyperactivity disorder (ADHD), psychomotor slowing (fine motor deficits that may impair writing and speech), and worsening of ADHD combined with conduct disorders (Belman, 1990; Belman et al., 1986). As the HIV-1 encephalopathy progresses, severe deficits in motor planning, speech, language, and cognition are to be expected.

Limited data are available on the neuropsychological performance differences of asymptomatic, mildly symptomatic, or older children with early or late stage HIV-1 CNS disease. Belman (1992) reported a study of children who were exposed to HIV-1 through blood transfusion during the neonatal period. The group was divided into seropositive and seronegative children. At the time of the study, 67% of the seropositive children were asymptomatic. The two groups did not differ on the basis of overall intelligence quotients (IQ) test scores. However, small but significant differences were noted on various subtests of motor speed, visual scanning, and cognitive flexibility. This finding is in agreement with results from a similar study (Diamond et al., 1987). These studies suggest that the two domains of mental function that are most affected by HIV-1 are expressive language and attention.

A consistent finding in school-aged children with HIV-1 infection is that very few will perform in the normal range on standardized cognitive assessment instruments (Diamond et al., 1990). Cognitive deficits are evident in decreased intellectual levels, specific learning disabilities, mental retardation, visual-spatial deficits, and decreased alertness.

Acquired microcephaly is common in children with HIV-1-related encephalopathy (Belman, 1992; Jenkins, 1996; Wiznia et al., 1996). This reduced head circumference is due to calcification of the brain's white matter and basal ganglia. Changes in, or loss of, white matter results in deficits in short-term memory, speed of processing, visual-motor coordination, and sequencing abilities (Brouwers et al., 1991; Cousens, Ungerer, Crawford, & Stevens, 1991).

In addition to specific neurodevelopmental deficits and delays, social and behavioral problems are evident in preschool and school-aged children who were perinatally infected with HIV-1 (Seidel, 1991). These problems may exist due to HIV-1 involvement in the frontal cortex, basal ganglia, and connecting structures in the CNS (Belman, 1990). These structures have been associated with regulation of attention and concentration, and in some cases, other emotional behaviors in children (Tramontana & Hooper, 1989). Behavioral and emotional problems also may exist as a result of multiple stressors in the lives of children with HIV-1 infection. Attention deficits, hyperactivity, depression, and anxiety may be due to a parent's death or illness, chaotic family environment, poverty, prenatal exposure to drugs, or premature birth (Anastos, Denenberg, & Solomon, 1997; Barkley, 1990; Kletter et al., 1989; Marcus et al., 1989).

The prevalence of ADHD in children with HIV-1 infection is relatively high, especially in children who, in addition to exposure to HIV-1, were exposed in utero to drugs or born prematurely (Belman, 1992; DePaul & Barkley, 1990; Lifschitz, Hanson, Wilson, & Shearer, 1989; Moss et al., 1989; Moss et al., 1990). At this time, it is unclear if disorders of attention in infected children can be attributed to HIV-1 infection, other factors such as discussed above, or a combination of both.

Identification of factors that produce behavioral problems in children with HIV-1 infection is critical to intervention strategies (Seidel, 1991). If the problems are due to CNS involvement by HIV-1, then a physician will need to treat the problem medically. However, if the problems are due to environmental factors, then behavioral intervention strategies may be beneficial in reducing the negative behaviors.

HIV-1 disease remains incurable, but recent advances in antiretroviral agents and better management of medical symptoms have increased life expectancy in the pediatric HIV-1-infected population. With extended life-span, more children will be attending school. School systems will be faced with developing programs to meet the needs of these children with developmental, learning, behavioral, and communication disorders. It is important to recognize that many children have multiple deficits and will require interdisciplinary services.

Psychosocial Factors

It is very important to consider the impact of the maternal and home environment when interpreting study results of neurocognitive and behavioral functioning in children with HIV-1. In one pediatric AIDS developmental program, it was reported that only 20 to 25% of these children lived at home with their biological family (Hopkins, 1989). The majority resided in foster care (55 to 60%) or lived with relatives and unrelated caretakers (20 to 25%). A small percentage of infected children were institutionalized. According to Hopkins, children who were in foster care or institutionalized were found to be at greater risk for cognitive deficits later in life than those who lived with their biological parents.

A longitudinal study of the children of women who were infected with HIV-1 found a significant relationship among overall child development, the quality of the mother-child relationship, and socioeconomic status (Condrini et al., 1993). The study concluded that no correlation was found between HIV status and intelligence. The results suggest that child development is related more to socioeconomic status and maternal factors than to clinical status.

CHAPTER SUMMARY

The course of HIV-1 infection is similar in adults and children. However, there are several notable differences. Some of the most important distinctions are:

- perinatally exposed children experience more rapid disease progression
- chronic respiratory and pulmonary disease affect the pediatric population more than in adult infection
- lymphoid interstitial pneumonitis and recurring bacterial infections appear unique to pediatric AIDS
- small size for gestational age, acquired microcephaly
- failure to thrive
- recurrent bacterial pneumonia or infections, which are unique to pediatric HIV-1

- certain opportunistic infections (*Cryptococcus,* toxoplasmosis, cytomegalovirus, and Kaposi's sarcoma) that are so prevalent in adults are less common in children
- recurrent otitis media, sinusitis, mastoiditis
- *Pneumocystis carinii* pneumonia (PCP) and encephalopathy occur early in children who demonstrate rapid disease progression (rapid progressors)
- hepatosplenomegaly (enlarged liver and spleen)
- lymphadenopathy (enlarged lymph nodes)
- chronic oral candidiasis and esophagitis causing dysphagia and odynophagia

School-aged children with pediatric HIV-1 exhibit a variety of motor, speech, language, hearing, and cognitive deficits that present an educational challenge. Attention deficit disorder and behavioral problems may also complicate the educational process.

Developmental delays are found frequently in children with HIV-1 (Armstrong, Seidel, & Swales, 1993; Belman; 1992; Brouwers et al., 1991; Pressman, 1992; Seidel, 1991). However, caution must be used in drawing a cause-and-effect relationship between HIV-1 status and developmental delays. It is notable that a relatively high incidence of developmental delays occur in children who are not infected with HIV-1 born to women who are infected. Other factors such as prematurity, prenatal exposure to drugs and alcohol, and poor prenatal care all may be contributing factors to the deficits (Kletter et al., 1989; Marcus et al., 1989; Pressman, 1992; Swales, 1991).

7

Counseling Issues

It is realized that speech-language pathologists and audiologists are not trained to be professional counselors. When profound emotional and psychological disturbances are observed in their clients, clinicians need to be quick in making referrals to trained mental health professionals. However, it can be expected that, as rapport between the clients and their clinicians grows, clients will confide or reveal their fears in the course of therapy. Having some understanding of the emotional and psychological strain caused by the knowledge of being HIV-1 positive will give clinicians added insight. Such an understanding will better prepare clinicians to handle their clients' emotional expressions appropriately.

This chapter will present information to aid the speech-language pathologist and audiologist in the difficult task of counseling an individual with HIV-1. Communication disorders specialists can also serve as excellent referral sources to other services and support groups available to persons with HIV-1 and their families or significant others. This chapter includes governmental and community resources for clinicians and their clients to use.

ISSUES IN PROVIDING CARE FOR PEOPLE WITH HIV-1

The management of individuals with HIV-1 infection presents many clinical, physical, and emotional challenges for clinicians. Those individuals in the highest risk groups, including intravenous drug users, male homosexuals, and prostitutes, may be especially lacking in family and social support. The frightening prospect of progressive debilitation, social isolation, and death causes patients with HIV-1 infection to frequently turn to their care-providers for emotional support and reassurance.

People with HIV-1 have widely different experiences with the amount and quality of care they receive. In the early days of the disease, there was greater fear of caring for an infected person due to the lack of solid research on which body fluids transmitted the virus. In some cases, the clinician's fear for personal safety impeded the clinician-client relationship. As research findings increased, education of those who work with this population has been successful in changing negative attitudes and decreasing fear of transmission through routine contact. Nonetheless, even though the chances of healthcare workers becoming infected are slight, the threat is always present.

Fear of infection is not the only stress associated with caring for people with HIV-1 infection. Most people who are infected are young and may even be children. As these patients decline physically, the clinician also observes the psychological and emotional effects of the disease. Many patients and their significant others are on a roller-coaster ride of hopes and fears. All humans are interconnected and it is difficult to see the suffering of another and not be personally affected as a result.

Counseling is a part of case management but clinicians must never exceed the limits of their professional ability in counseling. As communication disorders professionals, we are not trained to effectively counsel serious depression, persistent anxiety, uncontrollable anger, or other symptoms of serious psychological duress. The client with HIV-1 infection often will be receiving counseling through social services. If not, these clients must always be referred to such professional counselors as psychiatrists, psychologists, clergymen, or social workers.

Emotional and Psychological Toll of HIV-1 Infection

Those who learn that they are infected with a deadly virus experience a wide range of strong emotions. Nearly everyone is likely to experience feelings of anger, depression, fatigue, fear, anxiety, and guilt. These feelings do not occur in predictable stages or intensity. Some people are overwhelmed by several or all the feelings at once.

Anger is a natural and justifiable response to this infection. People need to be allowed to be angry. To deal appropriately with this anger, the person must learn to express it in a constructive, not destructive, manner. Anger turned inward results in depression and self-damaging behavior. Anger turned outward causes the individuals to lash out at caregivers or significant others in their lives.

The first step in appropriately expressing anger is to separate the anger from the target. The clinician should help the individual identify the real cause of his or her anger. Generally, individuals infected with HIV-1 are angry at the uncontrollable circumstances in their lives. Second, the clinician should identify mechanisms that constructively discharge anger. Different methods work for different people. Examples of actions that help alleviate anger include rigorous physical exercise, meditation and relaxation techniques, keeping a journal about personal experiences, or finding a quiet place to scream and yell. Properly channeling anger releases much energy the individual can then use to accomplish productive things.

Another common emotion experienced by individuals is depression. Depression may be mild or severe. Mild depression basically runs its course within a few days and often resolves itself without intervention. To help dispel mild depression, the clinician should suggest increased social interaction, more physical exercise, occupying the mind with such activities as reading or watching a movie, or doing something that brings a sense of accomplishment. This may come from doing something small like cleaning out a closet, writing a letter, or baking cookies for someone else. No matter how small, the sense of accomplishment will often lift the spirit above depression.

When depression lasts too long or overwhelms the individual, professional help is indicated. Signs of severe depression include feelings of alienation, deep apathy, profound hopelessness, and chronic lethargy. Severe, persistent depression may require medication to combat it. In the case of an individual with AIDS or HIV-1 infection, the cause of severe depression is an understandable reaction to having a fatal disease. These individuals need a proper support network and medication under a professional's care.

Fatigue often accompanies depression. To compound the problem, fatigue also is an indirect consequence of HIV-1 infection (Bartlett & Finkbeiner, 1993). Other physical factors contribute to depression. For example, metabolic imbalances are a common problem in those with HIV-1. These imbalances cause anemia, fatigue, diarrhea, and cognitive changes, and are frequently accompanied by weight loss, fever, and night sweats. These symptoms most often occur late in the course of infection.

HIV-1 infection causes fatigue by depriving the body of some of its sources of energy through anemia and diarrhea. Anemia is a common finding among people with HIV-1, resulting in a lower number of red blood cells. One of the functions of red blood cells is to supply oxygen to cells. This oxygen then supplies muscles with energy. Although the causes of fatigue are physical, the effects are psychological. Fatigue may bring on depression, and vice versa.

Another finding in many persons with HIV-1 is chronic diarrhea. This condition causes food to pass through the body too quickly, not allowing sufficient nutrients to be absorbed, and the body is unable to derive energy from the food. This leads to malnutrition and dehydration which, in turn, leads to fatigue and cognitive changes.

A person with HIV-1 experiences both rational and irrational fears. Fear can be a paralyzing emotion. People fear most what they do not know or understand. For the person diagnosed with HIV-1, there are many unknown and uncontrollable variables. Such lack of information creates fear and anxiety in the majority of people with the virus. Persistent anxiety can be treated with medication or through the use of relaxation techniques taught by mental health professionals. If the patient is afraid of dying, counseling by a clergyman may provide some peace of mind.

An effective tool to dissipate the fear of the unknown is to gain information about what is feared. Clinicians can provide information about the disease, its treatment, available support groups, and other relevant information to ease the fears. By being informed, the clinician can serve as a valuable referral resource to clients.

One final debilitating emotion that many people who are HIV-1 positive feel is guilt: guilt for having become infected, guilt for bringing HIV infection into the lives of other people, guilt about the behavior that placed them at risk in the first place. Even those who contracted AIDS through means that society does not condemn, such as blood transfusions or hemophilia, express guilt.

Guilt, like fear, is an emotion that may not be based on facts. However, it is important to remember that guilt, like all the other emotional reactions to HIV-1 infection, is a natural human feeling. Guilt may stem from the belief that good behavior deserves rewards and bad behavior deserves punishment. Because dying from a virus is like a punishment, people feel that they must have done something wrong to be punished. To compound this guilt feeling, initial societal response to AIDS was that most people infected by the virus got what they deserved. Although society has become more sensitive to the issues surrounding infection, a certain amount of social stigma still remains.

Clinicians can assist their clients by helping them to separate the virus from a sense of punishment. The virus has nothing to do with punishment. A virus does not have a built-in mechanism to determine who is worthy of being spared or deserves to be infected. A virus has no value system and is not judgmental. It is simply a virus.

Clinicians should help the client who is infected to realize that guilt is an emotion that is harmful and nonproductive. Guilt causes the person to waste energy worrying about something he or she cannot change. Clinicians should help their clients to see that they are not just HIV-1-infected persons. They are persons with HIV-1 infection. It is important to point out that they have many characteristics that are good and valuable. Therefore, clinicians should help these clients focus on those aspects of their lives so they are able to counteract or attenuate guilt by understanding their own worth.

It is worth reiterating that if the client needs more counseling than the clinician can provide, the client should be referred to qualified counselors. Even clinicians who do not provide counseling to any significant extent should have a thorough understanding of the emotional reactions of persons with HIV-1. Such an understanding is essential for making a valid assessment of the communication needs of people with HIV-1. If clients are unable to communicate effectively, it will be more difficult for them to face, clarify, and possibly modify their complex emotional reactions. Therefore, helping them acquire effective communication skills to properly address their emotional reactions may be a service that communication disorders specialists can provide to these patients.

Improving Communication Skills

Communication is a two-way process between a speaker and a listener. In an interaction between two people, each takes turns being a speaker and a listener. Listening is probably the most important communication skill. Most people are much better at talking than they are at listening. Good listening requires effort to hear and understand what the speaker is saying and feeling. If the speaker was not clear in his or her communication, the listener must then ask for more information or clarification. Therefore, it is recommended that the skills of careful listening and asking specific questions to seek clarification be targeted in therapy.

Good communication skills are essential to persons who suffer from chronic illnesses. To receive good care, such persons must be able to adequately relay to doctors and other healthcare workers their medical concerns. In addition, effective communication is needed to ease the strained interpersonal relationships that often result from the illness. Poor communication is the biggest factor in poor relationships, whether the relationship is between spouses, family members, friends, or between doctor and patient. In therapy, communication disorder specialists should teach their clients to listen carefully and express specific ideas effectively.

One effective way to teach a new skill is for the clinician to model the desired behavior. Therefore, during counseling, it is very important that the clinician be a good listener. When the client speaks in generalities, the clinician should ask for more information. The clinician should paraphrase what was said to determine if that is what was actually meant. If more information is needed, the clinician should be specific in the questions asked to get that information. In this way, the clinician can obtain an accurate idea of what the client's needs are and how best to meet those needs.

Issues in Pediatric AIDS

Children living and coping with the myriad of stresses associated with having HIV-1 infection often experience indirect psychological effects.

These may include fear, anxiety, and emotional and behavioral reactions. Children infected with HIV-1 or AIDS have constant reminders that they are different from their peers, which is an added source of stress.

Children may be ostracized, rejected, and humiliated by peers if their illness becomes public knowledge. This may result in a sense of shame, guilt, and decreased self-esteem. In order to avoid the potential humiliation, disgrace, and persecution over being exposed, children with AIDS may hide their HIV status. This attempt to conceal their disease may result in withdrawal from friends and age-appropriate activities.

Most school-age children are aware that they have AIDS and that this is a fatal disease. At a young age, they experience living with a life-threatening disease, frequently witnessing the loss of other HIV-1-infected children they have come to know, and possibly, the loss of other family members. Younger children may be anxious about death because they perceive it as an event that separates them from family, loved ones, and friends. This separation anxiety may be reduced for some children by a family belief system that includes a belief in an afterlife in which one is reunited with loved ones.

Some children may express their distress by exhibiting hyperactivity and attentional deficit that are sufficient to interfere with school performance (Tramontana & Hooper, 1989). Attentional problems and hyperactivity may be an expression of the chronic unremitting tension that these children experience (Barkley, 1990). Children with HIV-1 or AIDS may exhibit periods of sadness and apparent depression. In general, behavioral problems are not extreme or incapacitating. However, more severe withdrawal behaviors sometimes occur early in childhood, some of which have been labeled "autistic-like" (Seidel, 1991).

Individual personalities dictate children's responses to the stresses of HIV-1 and AIDS. The effects on individual children vary as a function of the age of the child, the available support systems, the child's adaptive resources, and specific life circumstances. These circumstances include factors such as the number of other family members who are HIV-1-infected, socioeconomic status, drug dependency of a parent, and the nature of the family structure.

The majority of children with HIV-1 infection do not live in a traditional family structure. For example, one study reported only 20 to 25% of children infected with HIV-1 lived at home with their biological family (Hopkins, 1989). The majority resided in foster care (55 to 60%) or with relatives or unrelated caretakers (20 to 25%). A small percentage of pediatric AIDS patients are institutionalized.

The families of children with HIV-1 or AIDS often have fewer economic resources than other families, have minimal education, are unemployed, are single-parent families, are welfare-dependent, and have more than one family member affected by the disease (Seidel & Seibert, 1990).

The progression of AIDS in the child and other family members, poverty, and the effects of intravenous drug abuse by a parent are all challenging problems. The basic physical and emotional needs of these children often go unmet and commonly lead to foster care (Hopkins, 1989).

Parents of perinatally infected children may experience guilt over infecting their child. Combined with intravenous drug addiction, unemployment, lack of social support, and HIV-1-related psychiatric symptoms, these emotional responses may lead to significant maladaptive coping. All of these factors result in limited effectiveness in parenting a sick child. In extreme cases, the child's safety and welfare may be in jeopardy, requiring the involvement of child welfare services (Emery, Anderson, & Annin, 1992).

It is important to understand the range of the parent's or child's feelings and how this affects his or her ability to seek help. By acquiring a basic knowledge of some of the challenges that face children with AIDS and their families, the clinician will be more effective in treatment and as a referral source to needed information and services.

REFERENCE GUIDE OF SOURCES
FOR AIDS INFORMATION

Many needs of a client will be outside the speech-language pathologist's or audiologist's capabilities or domain of expertise. These clinicians will have to depend on other sources and professionals to obtain needed information or services for their clients. Therefore, clinicians should have a thorough knowledge about the various resources the patients can turn to.

The following is an extensive listing of government, national, state, and local organizations that provide information relevant to persons with HIV-1 infection and care providers. Before referring a patient to a source or an organization, the clinician should check the current address and telephone numbers as these may have changed subsequent to the publication of this book.

Centers for Disease Control and Prevention

The **Centers for Disease Control and Prevention (CDC)** has been working to inform people throughout the United States about HIV/AIDS since 1987. CDC has created a multiphase public education campaign and an organized information delivery system consisting of the CDC National AIDS Hotline and the CDC National AIDS Clearinghouse (CDC NAC). Staff members from these two programs respond to questions from the public and professionals on all aspects of HIV infection, from prevention and research to health care and support services.

The CDC NAC publishes a catalog with materials for health care providers, educators, policy makers, librarians, community-based organizations, and people living with HIV infection. Confidential information, referrals, and educational material on AIDS are available from the CDC National AIDS Hotline. NAC FAX is a service that allows people to obtain information directly via a fax machine. Selected documents, including CDC fact sheets, surveillance report tables, and information on Clearinghouse services are available free through the service

The CDC NAC offers a variety of Internet services including a World Wide Web site, a listserv of AIDS-related news, file transfer protocol (FTP), and gopher. The Web site contains information about Clearinghouse services, allows users to read the current AIDS Daily Summary and search back issues, and provides links to other Web and gopher sites. The listserv uses an automated mailing list to send electronic read-only HIV-related messages to subscribers. The FTP site allows users to download current information on HIV-1/AIDS without an individual password. The gopher system provides a simple menu which enables users to find documents and use with other Clearinghouse Internet services.

CDC National AIDS Clearinghouse
Mailing address:
CDC National AIDS Clearinghouse
P. O. Box 6003
Rockville, MD 20849-6003

Telephone: Monday through Friday, 9:00 a.m. to 7 p.m., eastern time.
1-800-458-5231 (Voice)
1-800-243-7012 (Deaf access/TDD)
1-301-251-5343 (Fax)

NAC FAX: Available 24 hours a day, 7 days a week.
1-800-458-5231 (Voice)

Internet resources:
E-mail: aidsinfo@cdcnac.aspensys.com
Web site: http://cdcnac.aspensys.com:86
Gopher: gopher://cdcnac.aspensys.com:72
Listserv: listserv@cdcnac.aspensys.com
FTP: ftp://cdcnac.aspensys.com/pub/cdcnac

CDC National AIDS Hotline
Telephone: 24 hours per day, 7 days per week, 365 days per year
1-800-342-AIDS (Voice)

1-800-344-7432 (Spanish access)
1-800-243-7889 (Deaf access/TTY)

HIV/AIDS Treatment Information Service
Provides federally approved treatment guidelines for HIV-1 and AIDS for health care providers and people living with HIV-1 infection.
1-800-448-0440 (Voice)

AIDS Clinical Trials Information Service
Provides up-to-date information on clinical trials that evaluate experimental drugs and other therapies for adults and children at all stages of HIV-1 infection.
1-800-TRIALS-A or 1-800-874-2572

National Organizational Contacts

ACT UP (nationwide information) .... (215) 731-1844
American Foundation for AIDS Research .... (202) 331-8600
Gay and Lesbian Alliance Against Defamation .... (212) 807-1700
Gay Men's Health Crisis AIDS Hotline .... (212) 807-6655
Indian AIDS Hotline .... (800) 283-2437
National Association of People with AIDS .... (202) 898-0414
National Hemophilia AIDS Foundation .... (800) 424-2634
National Lesbian and Gay Health Association .... (202) 939-7880
National Minority AIDS Council .... (202) 483-6622
National Women's Health Network .... (202) 347-1140
People with AIDS Coalition Hotline .... (800) 828-3280
People with AIDS Health Group .... (212) 255-0520
Project Inform Treatment Hotline .... (800) 822-7422
Spanish Information Hotline (SIDA) .... (800) 344-7432

State AIDS Hotline

Alabama	(800) 228-0469	Montana	(800) 233-6668
Alaska	(800) 478-2437	Nebraska	(800) 782-2437
Arizona	(602) 265-3300	Nevada	(800) 842-2437
Arkansas	(800) 364-2437	New Hampshire	(800) 842-2437
California, north	(800) 367-2437	New Jersey	(800) 624-2377
California, south	(800) 922-2437	New Mexico	(800) 545-2437
Colorado	(800) 252-2437	New York	(800) 872-2777
Connecticut	(800) 203-1234	New York	(800) 541-2437
Delaware	(800) 422-0429	North Carolina	(800) 342-2437

District of Columbia	(202) 332-2437	North Dakota	(800) 472-2180
Florida	(800) 352-2437	Ohio	(800) 332-2437
Georgia	(800) 551-2728	Oklahoma	(800) 535-2437
Hawaii	(800) 922-1313	Oregon	(800) 777-2437
Idaho	(208) 345-2277	Pennsylvania	(800) 662-6080
Illinois	(800) 243-2437	Puerto Rico	(809) 765-1010
Indiana	(800) 848-2437	Rhode Island	(800) 726-3010
Iowa	(800) 445-2437	South Carolina	(800) 322-2437
Kansas	(800) 232-0040	South Dakota	(800) 592-1861
Kentucky	(800) 654-2437	Tennessee	(800) 525-2437
Louisiana	(800) 922-4379	Texas	(800) 299-2437
Maine	(800) 851-2437	Utah	(800) 366-2437
Maryland	(800) 638-6152	Vermont	(800) 882-2437
Massachusetts	(800) 235-2331	Virgin Islands	(809) 773-2437
Michigan	(800) 872-2437	Virginia	(800) 533-4148
Minnesota	(800) 248-2437	Washington	(800) 272-2437
Mississippi	(800) 826-2961	West Virginia	(800) 642-8244
Missouri	(800) 533-2437	Wisconsin	(800) 334-2437
Montana	(800) 233-6668	Wyoming	(800) 327-3577

State Prescription-Drug Assistance Programs

State financial assistance is available and can be an excellent source of other benefits for people with HIV-1 infection and AIDS. The individual needs a prescription from a physician or an application showing his or her HIV status and financial qualification. Individuals may call the following numbers to find out what is available in their state.

Alabama	(334) 613-5364	Montana	(406) 444-4744
Alaska	N/A	Nebraska	(402) 559-4673
Arizona	(602) 230-5819	Nevada	(702) 687-4800
Arkansas	(501) 376-6299	New Hampshire	(800) 852-3345
California, north	(800) 858-2437	New Jersey	(609) 588-7038
California, south	(800) 858-2437	New Mexico	(800) 545-2437
Colorado	N/A	New York	(800) 872-2777
Connecticut	(800) 233-2503	North Carolina	(919) 733-3091
Delaware	(302) 995-8653	North Dakota	(701) 328-2378
District of Columbia	(202) 347-8888	Ohio	(614) 466-6669
Florida	(904) 922-6675	Oklahoma	(800) 285-2273
Georgia	(404) 657-3129	Oregon	(503) 731-4029
Hawaii	(808) 732-0315	Pennsylvania	(800) 922-9384
Idaho	(208) 334-6657	Puerto Rico	(809) 765-1010
Illinois	(800) 825-3518	Rhode Island	(401) 464-2183
Indiana	(317) 920-3190	South Carolina	(800) 856-9954
Iowa	(515) 242-5838	South Dakota	(800) 592-1861
Kansas	(913) 296-8891	Tennessee	(615) 741-8903

Kentucky	(502) 564-6539	Texas	(800) 255-1090
Louisiana	(504) 568-5304	Utah	(801) 538-6197
Maine	(207) 287-5060	Vermont	(800) 987-2839
Maryland	N/A	Virgin Islands	N/A
Massachusetts	(800) 228-2714	Virginia	(804) 225-4844
Michigan	(517) 335-9333	Washington	(800) 272-2437
Minnesota	(800) 657-3761	West Virginia	(304) 345-4673
Mississippi	(601) 960-7723	Wisconsin	(608) 267-6875
Missouri	(314) 751-6439	Wyoming	(307) 777-5800

Services for Ethnic and Minority Groups

African-Americans

American Red Cross, African-American HIV/
    AIDS Program .... (703) 206-7411
Black, Gay, and Lesbian Leadership Forum .... (213) 964-7820
Howard University, National AIDS Minority
    Information and Education Program .... (202) 865-3720
National Black Women's Health Project .... (404) 758-9590
National Task Force on AIDS Prevention .... (415) 356-8100

Asian-Pacific Islanders

Asian and Pacific Islander American Health
    Forum .... (415) 541-0866
Association off Asian-Pacific Community Health
    Organizations .... (510) 272-9536
National Asian-Pacific American Families
    Against Substance Abuse .... (213) 278-0031
Organization of Chinese American Women .... (202) 638-0330

Hispanics

American Red Cross, Hispanic HIV/AIDS
    Program .... (703) 206-7602
National Coalition of Hispanic Health and
    Human Services Organization .... (202) 387-5000
National Council of La Raza .... (202) 785-1670
National Puerto Rican Coalition .... (202) 223-3915

Native Americans

American Indian Health Care Association .... (800) 473-1926
National Congress of American Indians .... (202) 466-7767

National Native American AIDS Prevention
Center .... (510) 261-2505

Hearing- and Speech-Impaired

The following numbers are TTY/TDD numbers. The asterisk (*) indicates
a voice and TTY line so caller may need to tap the space bar to let them
know it is a TTY call.

AIDS Clinical Trial Information Service .... (800) 243-7012
AIDS Information Line .... (800) 551-2728
AIDS Project Inc. .... *(800) 851-2437
Business and Labor Respond to AIDS Resource
Service .... (800) 243-7012
CDC National AIDS Clearinghouse .... (800) 243-7012
Department of Medical Assistance Services .... (800) 343-0634
Disability Rights Center, Inc. .... (800) 834-1721
HIV/AIDS Treatment Information Service .... (800) 243-7012
National Association of People with AIDS .... *(202) 898-0414

Women

National Resource Center on Women
and AIDS .... (202) 872-1770
National Women's Health Resource Center .... (202) 293-6045
National Women's Health Network .... (202) 347-1140
Women's Information & Service Exchange .... (404) 817-3441
Women Organized to Respond to Life-
Threatening Diseases .... (510) 658-6930

General Ethnic and Minority

The Office of Minority Health .... (800) 444-6472
The National Minority AIDS Council .... (800) 559-4145

HIV/AIDS-related Publications

Publication	Address	Description
AIDS Treatment News	John S. James PO Box 411256 San Francisco, CA 94141 (800) 873-2812	Biweekly developments in research, experimental therapies, politics, and treatments are presented. $100/year or $60/6 months; (sliding scale available)

Body Positive	2095 Broadway Suite 306 New York, NY 10023 (212) 566-7333	Nontechnical monthly magazine for people who are HIV positive. Available in Spanish on a limited basis. Voluntary contributions accepted.
Critical Path AIDS Project	2062 Lombard Street Philadelphia, PA 19146 (215) 545-2212	AIDS Library of Philadelphia monthly. Specific medical news, social concerns, and some excerpts of interest from other publications. $50/year, free to people with AIDS.
HIV/AIDS Resources: The National Directory of Resources on HIV Infection/ AIDS	(800) 225-1860	Annual guide of nationwide services, education, prevention, hotlines and medical facilities for HIV/AIDS.
Notes from the Underground	PWA Health Group of NYC Buyers' Club 150 West 26th Street Suite 201 New York, NY 10001	Focus is on alternative therapies and "underground" treatments. Bimonthly. $75 to institutions, $35 to others, sliding scale for people with AIDS.
Positively Aware	Test Positively Aware Network 1340 West Irving Park Box 259 Chicago, IL 60613 (312) 472-6397	Published quarterly. Although written for the newly diagnosed person with HIV-1, the thematic issues are universally relevant.
The Positive Woman	PO Box 34372 Washington, DC 20043	Published every 2 months. Presents a mix of conventional and other therapy information, plus reader input, social issues and other issues from a woman's perspective. Written for mostly female audience.

PEDIATRIC RESOURCES *

*From Project Inform; for more information contact the Project Inform National HIV/AIDS Treatment Hotline, (800) 822-7422. Internet: http://www.projinf.org

CDC National AIDS Hotline

AIDS information and referrals, 24 hours a day, 7 days a week. 1-800-342-AIDS (2437).

Organizations

- **Association for the Care of Children's Health (ACCH):** Advocacy and education; organization of professionals and parents concerned with the needs of children in health care settings. 7910 Woodmont Ave., Suite 300, Bethesda, MD 20814. (301) 654-6549.
- **At-Risk Baby Crib (ABC) Quilts:** Provides free baby quilts and booties to HIV-positive newborns to 6 year olds. (603) 942-9211.
- **For AIDS Children Everywhere (FACE):** Offers emergency financial assistance, clothing, and emotional support to families in Cincinnati area. POB 46974, Cincinnati, OH 45246-0794. (513) 558-3571.
- **Families' and Children's AIDS Network (FCAN):** Works to meet the needs of families and children living with HIV/AIDS. Information, referral, educational forums, coordination of services among providers, and Network News newsletter. 721 North LaSalle St., Suite 311, Chicago IL 60610. Phone : (312) 655-7360. Fax: (312) 944-8906.
- **Foundation for Children with AIDS:** Services for families with HIV-positive children. Publications include a newsletter on programs and services for children with HIV or AIDS and their families. Information and referral about children with AIDS, series, and current literature. 1800 Columbus Ave., Roxbury, MA 02119. (617) 442-7442.
- **Just Kids Project of Three Corners Community Initiative:** Focuses on self-empowerment of parents and HIV-positive children, and getting more medical treatments available to children and adolescents. Publishes *Just Kids Newsletter.* Contact Emily Gordon, Just Kids Project, POB 42, New York, NY 10014. (212 627-3390. Fax: (212) 807-0347.

- **National Pediatric HIV Resource Center (NPHRC):** Provides consultation, training, and forum for exploring public policy issues related to pediatric AIDS. Organization has developed recommendations on the medical management of HIV-infected children. Contact NPHRC for publications list. NPHRC, 15 S. Ninth St., Newark, NJ 17107. (201) 268-8251 or (800) 362-0071. Fax (201) 485-2752.
- **Pediatric AIDS Foundation:** Raises money for pediatric AIDS research, provides information and referrals, emergency assistance to hospitals serving children with HIV and AIDS, sponsors educational programs and student internships. 1311 Colorado Ave., Santa Monica, CA 90404. (310) 395-9051.
- **Positively Pediatrics and Adolescents:** Provides education and support services for families, friends, and service providers of children and adolescents with HIV and AIDS. Speakers bureau to educate communities. POB 4512 Queensbury, NY 12804. (518) 798-8940.
- **Sunburst National AIDS Project:** Week-long residential camp for HIV-impacted families. Camp and transportation free to families. Medical care and counseling provided. 148 Wilson Hill Road, Petaluma, CA 94951. (707) 769-1269.

Foster Care and Adoption Programs

- **AID to Adoption of Special Kids:** Information on licensed adoption agencies. Help prospective families who wish to adopt children of parent with AIDS. 2201 Broadway, Oakland, CA 94612. (415) 543-2275.
- **Children with AIDS Project of America:** Helps match HIV-positive children and AIDS orphans with foster or adoptive families. POB 83131, Phoenix, AZ 85071-3131. (800) 866-2437.
- **National Adoption Information Clearinghouse:** Answers questions about adopting a child with HIV. (301) 231-6512.

Groups that Grant Wishes

- **Americans for Sound AIDS Policy (ASAP) Children's Christmas Fund:** Provides Christmas gifts for children with HIV infection. Contact: Anita Smith, POB 17433, Washington, DC 20041. (703) 471-7350.
- **Grant-A-Wish Foundation:** Grants wishes to children between 2½ and 18 years of age who have a life-threatening illness that

creates the probability that the child might not survive beyond his or her 18th birthday. 100 W. Clarendon #2200, Phoenix, AZ 85013. (800) 722-WISH (9474).

- **Starlite Foundation:** Grants wishes to critically, chronically, or terminally ill children, ages 4–18. 12233 W. Olympic Blvd. 322, Los Angeles, CA 90064. (800) 274-7827.

Glossary

acquired immunodeficiency syndrome (AIDS): Disease of the immune system in previously healthy individuals caused by infection with the human immunodeficiency virus (HIV).

acquired microcephaly: Reduction of head circumference in a previously normal-sized head. In children with HIV-1-associated encephalopathy, this reduction is due to calcification of the brain's white matter and basal ganglia.

acute infection of HIV-1: One to six weeks after transmission of HIV-1, an infectious mononucleosis-like illness develops. The individual recovers in one to two weeks, and some never notice this stage.

AIDS dementia complex (ADC): Dementia that occurs when the human immunodeficiency virus (HIV) directly infects the central nervous system.

anaphylaxis: An allergic hypersensitivity reaction of the body to a foreign substance or drug. Severe anaphylaxis may lead to anaphylactic shock, which may result in death if emergency treatment is not given.

antibodies: A protein substance the immune system produces in response to exposure to an antigen. The antibody interacts specifically with the antigen, which is the basis of immunity. It takes approximately four to twelve weeks for an adult to develop HIV-1 antibodies after exposure. Perinatally exposed infants may develop HIV-1 antibodies and test positive in 48 hours from birth if they were infected in utero (prenatally). If infected during the birth process, antibodies will be evident 7 to 90 days after birth.

antigen: Any substance introduced into the body or naturally formed within the body that causes the formation of antibodies that interact specifically with it. Examples of antigens are bacteria, toxins, foreign blood cells, and viruses.

apoptosis: Disintegration of cells into particles that are then ingested by phagocytes. Apoptosis is triggered by changes in the cellular environment that cause it to self-destruct. It is theorized that the presence of HIV-1 is cytotoxic, causing neurons to "commit suicide" by initiating apoptosis.

asymptomatic HIV-1 infection: A variable time interlude after seroconversion during which individuals feel well, function normally, and exhibit none of the HIV-1-related opportunistic infections or complications.

ataxia: Inability to coordinate or control voluntary motor movement.

attention deficit, hyperactivity disorder (ADHD): The American Psychiatric Association describes this as a disease of infancy and childhood, characterized by developmentally inappropriate inattention, impulsivity, and hyperactivity. The onset is usually by age three and the disorder is 10 times more common in boys than girls.

bilateral corticospinal tract signs: Indications of damage to the central nervous tract that allows nerve impulses to travel from the cerebral cortex and spinal cord. These signs include weakness or incoordination of upper extremities, lower extremities, or both, which may result in spasticity, gait disturbances, inability to bear weight, or maintenance of balance.

brain parenchyma: The essential parts of the brain concerned with its function (e. g., white matter, gray matter).

CC CKR 5: A cell membrane-bound protein that is a partner of CD4 (a coreceptor) in allowing HIV-1 to enter target cells in the critical early stages of infection

CD4 lymphocytes: A white blood cell or lymphocyte. HIV-1 primarily infects cells with CD4 cell-surface receptor molecules, using them to gain entry into immune cells. Once HIV-1 enters the cell, it destroys the host cell and disguises itself with the DNA of the dead cell. This is why the depletion of CD4 cells is an accurate measure of disease progression.

cerebrovascular accidents (CVAs): A general term applied to cerebrovascular conditions that occur due to ischemic or hemorrhagic lesions.

chemokines: Proteins that help bring about inflammatory responses. Research has shown that the presence of chemokines in cells suppresses the ability of HIV-1 to infect cells.

clinical trial: A carefully designed and implemented investigation of the effects of a drug administered to human subjects. The goal is to define clinical efficacy, side effects, contraindications, and so forth, of the substance.

clonus: Spasmodic alternation of muscular contraction and relaxation.

CMV retinitis: Inflamed condition of the retina as result of infection by cytomegalovirus. Symptoms include diminished vision, altered visual perception of size of objects, and progressive vision loss that may lead to blindness.

cytomegalovirus (CMV): CMV is the most common opportunistic viral pathogen affecting the CNS. CMV is a DNA herpes virus that becomes latent after primary infection in a person with normal immune response. When the immune system is suppressed, reactivation of the infection occurs.

cytopathic: Ability to injure or destroy cells.

cytotoxic: Destructive to cells.

dementia: Deteriorated mental status with absence or reduction of intellectual faculties due to organic brain disorder. Dementia is associated with more than 70 diseases, disorders, and metabolic disturbances.

demyelinization: Destruction or removal of the myelin sheath of a nerve, which results in slowed or disordered brain function.

dysphagia: Inability to swallow or difficulty during swallowing due to oral, pharyngeal, or esophageal disorders.

early symptomatic HIV-1 infection: A period when the first symptoms or complications that indicate weakening of the immune system, or immunosuppression, appear. These conditions were previously termed AIDS-related complex (ARC). This period typically lasts five to eight years.

encephalopathy associated with HIV-1: A neurologic disorder due to HIV-1 infection of the brain. In adults, HIV-1-related encephalitis is responsible for progressive dementia. In pediatric HIV-1, encephalitis causes loss of developmental milestones, acquired microcephaly, and a variety of other neurologic complications.

esophagitis: Inflammation of the esophagus.

exposed but uninfected (EU): A small percentage of people who have been exposed to HIV-1 but have somehow suppressed HIV-1's ability to destroy the immune system, even for as long as a decade. It is theorized that these individuals may have higher levels of chemokines, fewer fusin or CC CKR 5 receptors, or both.

failure to thrive: A general term to describe infants who do not grow or develop according to normal or expected rate.

fusin: A cell membrane protein that works in combination with CD4 cells as a receptor site that allows cells to fuse with the surface of HIV-1, which is a key step in the infection process. Fusin has been shown to infect T-lymphocyte cells at later stages of the disease.

hemianopsia: Blindness for half of the visual field in one eye or both.

hemiparesis: Weakness that affects half of the body.

hemophilia: A hereditary blood disease characterized by failure of blood to clot and abnormal bleeding.

herpes simplex virus (HSV): A common viral infection that causes cold sores and fever blisters in persons with an intact immune system. HSV

can cause encephalitis or aseptic meningitis in adults with immunosuppression and meningoencephalitis in infants with HIV-1 infection.

human immunodeficiency virus type 1 (HIV-1): The virus that causes
AIDS in humans.

hypoglycemia: Deficiency of sugar in the blood. A condition in which the
glucose in the blood is abnormally low, resulting in acute fatigue,
restlessness, malaise, marked irritability, mental disturbances, delir-
ium, coma, and possibly, death.

hyponatremia: Decreased concentration of sodium in the blood.

hypoxemia: Insufficient oxygenation of the blood.

indinavir: A protease inhibitor drug.

Kaposi's sarcoma: Malignant neoplasm of the skin. For some unknown
reason, homosexual men are especially prone to develop this disease.
The appearance of the skin growths is a reliable indicator of disease
progression towards AIDS.

lymphadenopathy: Enlarged lymph nodes.

lymphocyte: A lymph cell.

lymphoid interstitial pneumonitis (LIP): A chronic infiltration of the
lungs that severely impairs the quality of life for persons with HIV-1
infection. LIP is reported primarily in pediatric HIV-1 cases with only
a small number of cases reported among adults.

lymph nodes: Lymph nodes produce lymphocytes and monocytes, and
act as filters keeping particulate matter, especially bacteria, from gain-
ing entrance to the bloodstream.

malaise: Discomfort, uneasiness, or change of disposition that may be
indicative of infection.

meninges: The three membranes lining the spinal cord and brain; dura
mater, arachnoid, and pia mater.

meningitis: Inflammation of the membranes of the spinal cord or brain.

meningovascular syphilis: A form of neurosyphilis that involves the
meninges and vascular structures in the brain or spinal cord or both.

metastasize: Spread from one part of the body to another.

mucocutaneous: Mucous membrane to skin contact.

myelopathy: Any pathological condition of the spinal cord.

neoplasms: New and abnormal formation of tissue, such as a growth or
tumor.

neurosyphilis: A form of syphilis that infects the nervous system. CNS
involvement by syphilis may be manifest as asymptomatic infection,
acute syphilitic meningitis, cerebral arthritis, stroke, deafness, as well
as optic neuropathy (such as eye inflammation and swollen or damaged retinas).

nuchal rigidity: Stiff neck.

odynophagia: Pain during swallowing.

opportunistic infections: Infections caused by any organism, but especially fungal, parasitic, and bacterial, in which infection occurs due to

the opportunity afforded by the suppression of the immune system of the host.

oral candidiasis: An opportunistic infection caused by Candida albicans of the mouth or throat. Characterized by formation of white patches and ulcers visible in the oral cavity, frequently accompanied by fever and gastrointestinal inflammation.

oral hairy leukoplakia: This is the most common manifestation found in persons with HIV-1 infection and is caused by the Epstein-Barr virus. The development of this condition is a reliable indicator of subsequent development of AIDS in approximately 24 months from time of onset of oral hairy leukoplakia.

otalgia: Pain in the ear.

otorrhea: Discharge from the ear.

otosyphilis: A form of neurosyphilis that affects the inner ear.

percutaneous: Effected through the skin.

perinatal transmission: Transmission of HIV-1 from mother to child during the prenatal or in utero stage, during the child birth process, or shortly after birth in the neonatal stage.

pernicious anemia: A severe form of blood disease characterized by progressive decrease in red blood corpuscles, muscular weakness, and gastrointestinal and neural disturbances as a result of vitamin B12 deficiency. This is the most common nutritional deficiency in persons with HIV-1 infection.

phagocytes: Cells that have the ability to ingest and destroy particulate substances (e. g., bacteria, cell debris).

photophobia: Intolerance to light.

placebo: An inactive substance often used in a controlled study to determine the effects of a test substance.

Pneumocystis carinii **otitis media (PcOM):** This is an opportunistic bacterial infection of the middle ear unique to HIV-1 disease in children. Acute or recurrent otitis media may be due to bacterial infection of the respiratory tract by *Pneumocystis carinii.*

Pneumocystis carinii **pneumonia:** An opportunistic infection caused by a parasitic organism, *Pneumocystis carinii,* resulting in acute interstitial plasma cell pneumonia. This is the most common of all AIDS-related illnesses in the United States. Over half of all AIDS patients died of complications of this opportunistic infection in the early years of the AIDS epidemic. Preventative therapy and improved drugs have significantly decreased the number of deaths attributable to this infection.

polyneuropathy: Any noninflammatory disorder of peripheral nerves.

progressive encephalopathy: The CNS disease syndrome associated with pediatric AIDS is HIV-related encephalopathy. A small but significant number of children with encephalopathy will have the progressive type of disorder. The most frequent manifestations include developmental delays, loss of achieved developmental milestones, acquired microcephaly, progressive cognitive impairments, bilateral corticospinal tract signs, and ataxia. Disease progression may be very rapid and profound impairments and death may occur in only one to two months from diagnosis of progressive encephalopathy.

progressive multifocal leukoencephalopathy (PML): A progressive demyelinating disease of the central nervous system that is opportunistic in immune compromised individuals. PML is caused by the activation of a common papovavirus (a group of viruses important in causing viral-related cancer), the J. C. virus (JCV).

prophylactic intervention or therapy: Any agent or regimen that contributes to the prevention of infection and disease.

protease inhibitors: A class of drugs that block the activity of a protease enzyme needed for HIV-1 replication.

rapid progressors: A group of perinatally HIV-1-infected children who demonstrate disease symptoms with the first year of life and progress to AIDS by 5 years of age.

retroviruses: The common name for a family of RNA-containing tumor viruses, some of which cause sarcoma, lymphomas, leukemias, and AIDS. These viruses contain reverse transcriptase. HIV-1 is a retrovirus.

reverse transcriptase: An enzyme which enables retroviruses, such as HIV-1, to convert from an RNA to a DNA copy in order to disguise itself, thereby escaping the immune systems attack.

ritonavir: A protease inhibitor.

seroconversion: The condition when the blood test for the presence of antibodies to HIV-1 is positive.

slow progressors: These are a group of perinatally HIV-1-infected children who remain asymptomatic for a longer period of time, demonstrating more effective suppression of viral replication in the first year of life.

spasticity: Increased tone or contractions of muscles causing stiff and awkward movements.

subdural hematoma: A swelling or mass of blood located beneath the dura mater.

T-helper lymphocytes: A critical component of the immune system, these cells enhance the production of antibody-forming cells from B-lymphocytes. Research has revealed that T-helper cells are particularly vulnerable to HIV-1.

thrombocytopenia: An abnormal decrease in the number of blood platelets that places person at risk for internal hemorrhage, especially cerebral.

toxoplasmosis: An infection caused by an intracellular protozoan that rarely causes infection in a person with an intact immune system. It is the most frequent of the HIV-1-associated opportunistic infections. Infection occurs primarily via the oral route through ingestion of raw or undercooked meat, then remains latent until immunosuppression occurs in the host.

transient ischemic attack (TIA): Temporary interference with blood supply to the brain that causes symptoms of neurologic disturbance that last for only a few moments or several hours. After the TIA, no residual deficits are evident.

triangulation: A research method applied to social science research to enhance the external validity of a study. Triangulation is the act of bringing multiple sources of data together to corroborate, elaborate, or illuminate the phenomena under study. The purpose of triangulation is to seek convergence of results.

uremia: Toxic condition associated with renal insufficiency and kidney dysfunction.

varicella zoster virus (VZV): VZV causes chicken pox in children and zoster (shingles) in adults with intact immune systems. In persons with immunosuppression, VZV is associated with several neurologic syndromes.

viral load count (viremia): Number of HIV-1 in a specific measure of blood or body fluid.

virus: A minute organism visible only with an electron microscope that is a parasite that is dependent on nutrients inside host cells for its metabolic and reproductive needs. Viruses consist of a strand of ribonucleic acid (RNA) or deoxyribonucleic acid (DNA) but not both. HIV-1 consists of a strand of RNA.

wasting syndrome: A term used to describe the rapidly progressive nature of malnutrition that is unique to HIV-1 infection.

xerostomia: Dryness of mouth caused by decreased salivary production.

zidovudine: An antiretroviral drug used in the early treatment of HIV-1 infection and AIDS.

References

Adle-Biassette, H., Levy, Y., Colombel, M., Poron, F., Natchev, S., Keohane, C., & Gray, F. (1995). Neuronal apoptosis in HIV infection in adults. *Neuropathology & Applied Neurobiology, 21*(3), 218–227.

Afdhal, N. H. (1995). Gastrointestinal manifestations. In M. A. Sande & P. A. Volberding (Eds.), *The Medical Management of AIDS* (4th ed., pp. 146–159). Philadelphia, PA: W. B. Saunders.

Alkhatib, G., Combadiere, C., Broder, C. C., Feng, Y., Kennedy, P. E., Murphy, P. M., & Berger E. A. (1996). CC CKR 5: A RANTES, MIP-1α, MIP-1β receptor as a fusion cofactor for macrophage-tropic HIV-1. *Science, 272,* 1955–1958.

American Foundation for AIDS Research. (1995). *AIDS/HIV Treatment Directory: Vol. 7.* Opportunistic infections and related disorders.

Anastos, K., Denenberg, R., & Solomon, L. (1997). Human immunodeficiency virus in women. *Medical Clinics of North America, 81*(2), 533–553.

Anonymous. (1984). Needlestick transmission of HTLV-III from a patient infected in Africa. *Lancet, 2,* 1376.

Arendt, G., Maecker, H-P., Purrman, J., & Homberg, V. (1994). Control of posture in patients with neurologically asymptomatic HIV infection and patients with beginning HIV-1–related encephalopathy. *Archives of Neurology, 51*(12), 1232–1235.

Armstrong, F. D., Seidel, J. F., & Swales, T. P. (1993). Pediatric HIV infection: A neuropsychological and educational challenge. *Journal of Learning Disabilities, 26*(2), 92–103.

Auperin, I., Mikol, J., Oksenhendler, E., Thiebaut, J. B., Brunet, M., Dupont, B., & Morinet, F. (1994). Primary central nervous system malignant non-Hodgkin's lymphomas from HIV-infected and non-infected patients: Expression of cellular surface proteins and Epstein-Barr viral markers. *Neuropathology & Applied Neurobiology, 20*(3), 243–252.

Baltimore, D. L. (1997). *A concerted national effort to develop an AIDS vaccine.* 37th Interscience Conference on Antimicrobial and Chemotherapy

(ICAAC), September 28–October 1, 1997, Toronto, Ontario, Canada, Abstract S-34.

Barkley, R. A. (1990). Associated problems, subtyping, and etiologies. In R. A. Barkley (Ed.), *Attention deficit hyperactivity disorder: A handbook for diagnosis and treatment* (pp. 74–105). New York: Guilford Press.

Barnes, D. M. (1986). AIDS-related brain damage unexplained. *Science, 232,* 1091–1093.

Barre-Sinoussi, F., Chermann, J-C., Rey, F., Nugeyre, M. T., Chamaret, S., Gruest, J., Dauguet, C., Axler-Blin, C., Vezinet-Brun, F., Rouzioux, C., Rozenbaum, W., & Montagnier, L. (1983). Isolation of a T-lymphotrophic retrovirus form a patient at risk for acquired immune deficiency syndrome (AIDS). *Science, 220,* 868–871.

Bartlett, J. G., & Finkbeiner, A. K. (1993). *The guide to living with HIV infection: Developed at the Johns Hopkins AIDS clinic* (Rev. ed.). Baltimore, MD: Johns Hopkins University Press.

Battinelli, D. L., & Peters, E. S. (1995). Oral Manifestations. In H. Libman & R. A. Witzburg (Eds.), *HIV infection: A clinical manual* (2nd ed., pp. 74–83). Boston, MA: Little, Brown and Company.

Beach, R. S., Morgan, R., Wilkie, F., Mantero-Atienza, E., Blaney, N., Shor-Posner, G., Lu, Y., Eisdorfer, C., & Baum, M. K. (1992). Plasma vitamin B12 level as a potential cofactor in studies of human immunodeficiency virus type1-related cognitive changes. *Archives of Neurology, 49*(5), 501–506.

Belec, L., Georges, A. J., Vuillecard, E., Galin, E., & Martin, P. M. V. (1988). Peripheral facial paralysis indicating HIV infection. *Lancet, 2,* 1421–1422.

Belman, A. L. (1990). Neurologic syndromes associated with symptomatic human immunodeficiency virus infection in infants and children. In P. B. Kozlowski, D. A. Snider, O. M. Vietze, & H. M. Wisniewski (Eds.), *Brain in pediatric AIDS* (pp. 45–63). Basel, Switzerland: S. Karger.

Belman, A. L. (1992). Acquired immunodeficiency syndrome and the child's central nervous system. *Pediatric Clinics of North America, 39,* 691–714.

Belman, A. L., Lantos, G., Horoupian, D., Novick, B. E., Ultmann, M. H., Dickson, D. W., & Rubinstein, A. (1986). AIDS: Calcification of the basal ganglia in infants and children. *Neurology, 36,* 1192–1199.

Belman, A. L., Ultmann, M. H., Horoupian, D., Novick, B. E., Spiro, A. J., Rubinstein, A., Kurtzberg, D., & Cone-Wesson, B. (1985). Neurological complications in infants and children with acquired immune deficiency syndrome (AIDS). *Annals of Neurology, 18,* 560–566.

Belman, A. L., Ultmann, M. H., Novick, B. E., Horoupian, D., Lantos, G., Diamond, G., Dickson, D., & Rubinstein, A. (1986). CNS involvement in infants and children with AIDS. *Annals of Neurology, 18,* 560–566.

Berky, Z. T., Luciano, J., & James, W. D. (1992). Latex glove allergy: A survey of the US Army Dental Corp. *Journal of the American Medical Association (JAMA), 268*(19), 2695–2697.

Berry, C. D., Hooton, T. M., Collier, A. C., & Lukehart, S. A. (1987). Neurologic relapse after benzathine penicillin therapy for secondary syphilis in a patient with HIV infection. *New England Journal of Medicine, 316,* 1587–1589.

Bluestone, C. D., & Klein, J. O. (1996). Otitis media, atelectasis, and eustachian tube dysfunction. In C. D. Bluestone, S. E. Stool, & M. A. Kenna (Eds.), *Pediatric otolaryngology* (3rd ed., Vol. 1, pp. 388–582). Philadelphia: W. B. Saunders.

Borg, W. R., & Gall, M. D. (1989). *Educational Research: An introduction* (5th ed.). New York: Longman.

Brettler, D. B., Forsberg, A., Bolivar, E., Brewster, F., & Sullivan, J. (1990). Growth failure as a prognostic indicator for progression to acquired immunodeficiency syndrome in children with hemophilia. *Journal of Pediatrics, 117*(4), 582–588.

Brouwers, P., Belman, A. L., & Epstein, L. G. (1991). Central nervous system involvement: Manifestations and evaluation. In P. A. Pizzo & C. M. Wilfert (Eds.), *Pediatric AIDS: The challenge of HIV infection in infants, children, and adolescents* (pp. 318–335). Baltimore: Williams & Wilkins.

Bryson, Y. J. (1995). HIV clearance in infants—a continuing saga. *AIDS, 9,* 1373–1375.

Burger, H., Weiser, B., Robinson, W. S., Lifson, J., Engleman, E., Rouzioux, C., Brun-Vezinet, F., Barre-sinoussi, F., Montagnier, L., & Chermann, J-L. (1986). Transmission of lymphendenopathy-associated virus/human T lymphotropic virus type III in sexual partners: Seropositivity does not predict infectivity in all cases. *American Journal of Medicine, 81*(1), 5–10.

Cello, J. P. (1995). Gastrointestinal tract manifestations of AIDS. In M. A. Sande & P. A. Volberding (Eds.), *The Medical Management of AIDS* (4th ed., pp. 241–260). Philadelphia, PA: W. B. Saunders.

Centers for Disease Control. (1981a). Pneumocystis pneumonia—Los Angeles. *Morbidity and Mortality Weekly Report, 30*(21), 250–252.

Centers for Disease Control. (1981b). Kaposi's sarcoma and pneumonia among homosexual men—New York City and California. *Morbidity and Mortality Weekly Report, 30*(33), 305–308.

Centers for Disease Control. (1981c). Follow up on Kaposi's sarcoma and Pneumocystis pneumonia. *Morbidity and Mortality Weekly Report, 30*(33), 409–410.

Centers for Disease Control. (1982a). Persistent generalized lymphadenopathy among homosexual males. *Morbidity and Mortality Weekly Report, 31*(19), 249–252.

Centers for Disease Control. (1982b). Update on Kaposi's sarcoma and opportunistic infections in previously healthy persons—United States. *Morbidity and Mortality Weekly Report, 31*(31), 431–438.

Centers for Disease Control. (1982c). Update on acquired immune deficiency syndrome (AIDS)—United States. *Morbidity and Mortality Weekly Report, 31*(37), 507–514.

Centers for Disease Control. (1982d). Update on acquired immune deficiency syndrome (AIDS) among patients with hemophilia A. *Morbidity and Mortality Weekly Report, 31*(48), 644–652.

Centers for Disease Control. (1982e). Unexplained immunodeficiency in opportunistic infections in infant—New York, New Jersey, California. *Morbidity and Mortality Weekly Report, 31*(49), 665–667.

Centers for Disease Control. (1983). Acquired immunodeficiency syndrome (AIDS) update—United States. *Morbidity and Mortality Weekly Report, 32*(24), 309–311.

Centers for Disease Control. (1985). Update: Acquired immunodeficiency syndrome (AIDS)—United States. *Morbidity and Mortality Weekly Report, 34*(18), 245–248.

Centers for Disease Control. (1986). Classification system for human T-lymphotrophic virus type III/lymphadenopathy-associated virus infections. *Morbidity and Mortality Weekly Report, 35*(20), 334–349.

Centers for Disease Control. (1987). Recommendation for prevention of HIV transmission in health-care settings. *Morbidity and Mortality Weekly Report, 36*(Suppl.), 2S.

Centers for Disease Control. (1990). Public health service statement on management of occupational exposure to human immunodeficiency virus, including considerations regarding zidovudine postexposure uses. *Morbidity and Mortality Weekly Report, 39*(RR-1).

Centers for Disease Control. (1991). Nosocomial transmission of multidrug-resistant tuberculosis among HIV-infected persons—Florida and New York, 1988–1991. *Morbidity and Mortality Weekly Report, 40,* 21.

Centers for Disease Control. (1992a). 1993 revised classification system for HIV infection and expanded surveillance case definition for AIDS among adolescents and adults. *Morbidity and Mortality Weekly Report, 41,* 1–17.

Centers for Disease Control. (1992b). Surveillance for occupationally acquired HIV infection—United States, 1981–1992. *Morbidity and Mortality Weekly Report, 41,* 823–825.

Centers for Disease Control. (1994a). Zidovudine for the prevention of HIV transmission from mother to infant. *Morbidity and Mortality Weekly Report, 43,* 285–287.

Centers for Disease Control. (1994b). National serosurveillance summary results through 1992, Vol 3. *U.S. Department of Health & Human Services, Public Health Service, Atlanta.*

Centers for Disease Control. (1994c). Update: AIDS among women—United States, 1994. *Morbidity and Mortality Weekly Report, 44,* 81–86.

Centers for Disease Control. (1995a). Update: Acquired immunodeficiency syndrome (AIDS)—United States, 1994. *Morbidity and Mortality Weekly Report, 44*(4), 64–67.

Centers for Disease Control. (1995b). AIDS map. *Morbidity and Mortality Weekly Report, 44*(38), 719.

Centers for Disease Control. (1995c). First 500,00 AIDS cases—United States, 1995. *Morbidity and Mortality Weekly Report, 44*(46), 849–853.

Centers for Disease Control. (1995d). HIV seroconversion among health care workers. *Morbidity and Mortality Weekly Report, 44*(50), 929–933.

Centers for Disease Control. (1996a). Update: Mortality attributable to HIV infection among persons aged 25–44 years—United States, 1994. *Morbidity and Mortality Weekly Report, 45*(6), 121–126.

Centers for Disease Control. (1996b). *FDA approved drugs for HIV infection and AIDS-related conditions—January 15, 1996.* Bethesda, MD: CDC National AIDS Clearinghouse.

Centers for Disease Control. (1996c). AIDS map. *Morbidity and Mortality Weekly Report, 45*(15), 316.

Centers for Disease Control. (1996d). HIV/AIDS surveillance report. *Morbidity and Mortality Weekly Report, 8*(1), 15.

Centers for Disease Control. (1997). Update: Trends in AIDS incidence, deaths, and prevalence—United States, 1996. *Morbidity and Mortality Weekly Report, 46*, 165–173.

Chelbowski, R. T., Grosvenor, M. B., Bernhard, N. H., Morales, L. S., & Bulcavage, L. M. (1989). National status, gastrointestinal dysfunction, and survival in patients with AIDS. *American Journal of Gastroenterology, 84*(10), 1288–1293.

Chimelli, L., Rosember, S., Hahn, M. D., Lope, M. B. S., & Barretto Netto, M. (1992). Pathology of the central nervous system in patients infected with the human immunodeficiency virus (HIV): A report of 252 autopsy cases from Brazil. *Neuropathology & Applied Neurobiology, 18*(5), 478–488.

Chin, J. (1994) The growing impact of the HIV/AIDS pandemic on children born to HIV infected women. *Clinical Perinatology, 21*, 1–15.

Ciardi, A., Sinclair, E., Scaaravilli, F., Harcourt-Webster, N., & Lucas, S. (1990). The involvement of cerebral cortex in human immunodeficiency virus encephalopathy: A morphological and immunohistochemical study. *Acta Neuropathologica, 81*(1), 51–59.

Cocchi, F., DeVico, A. L., Garzino-Demo, A., Arya, S. K., Gallo, R. C., & Lusso. (1995). Identification of RANTES, MIP-1α, MIP-1β as the major HIV-suppressive factors produced by CD8+ T cells. *Science, 270*, 1811–1815.

Cohen, J. (1996). Results on new AIDS drugs bring cautious optimism. *Science, 271*(9), 755–756.

Collier, A. C., Coombs, R. W., Schoenfeld, D. A., Bassett, R. L., Timpone, J., Baruch, A., Jones, M., Facey, K., Whitacre, C., McAuliffe, V. J., Friedman, H. M., Merigan, T. C., Reichman, R. C., Hooper, C., & Corey, L. (1996). Treatment of human immunodeficiency virus infection with saquinavir, zidovudine, and zalcitabine. *New England Journal of Medicine, 334*(16), 1011–1017.

Condrini, , A., Cattalan, C., Viero, F., Caella, S., Zampion, M., & Laverda, A. M. (1989). Psychic development of children born to HIV infected Italian mothers. *V International Conference on AIDS: Abstracts, 5*, 316.

Connor, E. M., Sperling, R. S., Gelber, R., Kiselev, P., Scott, G., O'Sullivan, M. J., Van Dyke, R., Bey, M., Shearer, W., Jacobson, R. L., Jimenez, E., O'Neill, E., Bazin, B., Delfraissy, J-F., Culnane, M., Coombs, R., Elkins, M., Meye, J., Stratton, P., & Belsley, J. for the Pediatric AIDS Clinical Trial Group protocol 076 study group. (1994). Reduction of maternal-infant transmission of human immunodeficiency virus Type 1infection with zidovudine treatment. *New England Journal of Medicine, 331*(18), 1173–1180.

Cousens, P., Ungerer, J. A., Crawford, J. A., & Stevens, M. M. (1991). Cognitive effects of childhood leukemia therapy: A case for specific deficits. *Journal of Pediatric Psychology, 16,* 475–488.

Creagh-Kirk, T., Doi, P., Andrews, E., Nusinoff-Lehrman, S., Tilson, H., Hroth, D, & Barry, D. (1988). Survival experience among patients with AIDS receiving zidovudine: Follow-up of patients in a compassionate plea program. *Journal of the American Medical Association (JAMA), 260*(20) 3009–3015.

Cruz, G. D., Lamster, I. B., Begg, M. D., Phelan, J. A., Gorman, J. M., & El-Sadr, W. (1996). The accurate diagnosis of oral lesions in human immuno-deficiency virus infection. *Archives of Otolaryngology Head & Neck Surgery, 122,* 68–73.

Deng, H. K., Liu, R., Ellmeier, W., Choe, S., Unatmaz, D., Burkhart, M., Di-Marzio, P., Marmon, S., Sutton, R. E., Hill, C, C. M., Davis, C. B., Peiper, S. C., Schall, T. J., Littman, D. R., & Landau, N. R. (1996). Identification of a major co-receptor for primary isolates of HIV-1. *Nature, 318,* 661–666.

DePaul, G. J., & Barkley, R. A. (1990). Medication therapy. In R. A. Barkley (Ed.), *Attention deficit hyperactivity disorder: A handbook for diagnosis and treatment* (pp. 573–612). New York: Guilford Press.

Diamond, G. W., Gurdin, P., Wiznia, A. A., Belman, A. L., Rubenstein, A., & Cohen, H. L. (1990). Effects of congenital HIV infection on neurodevelop-mental status of babies in foster care. *Developmental Medicine and Child Neurology, 32,* 999–1005.

Diamond, G. W. (1989). Developmental problems in children with HIV infec-tion. *Mental Retardation, 27,* 213–217.

Diamond, G. W., & Cohen, H. J. (1992). Developmental disabilities in children with HIV infection. In A. C. Crocker, H. J. Cohen, & T. A. Kastner (Eds.), *HIV infection and developmental disabilities: A resource for service providers* (pp. 33–42). Baltimore: Brookes.

Dichtel, W. J., Jr. (1992). Oral manifestations of human immunodeficiency virus infection. *Otolaryngologic Clinics of North America, 25*(6), 1211–1226.

DiPerri, G., Cruciani, M., Danzi, M. C., Luzzati, R., DeChecci, G., Malena, M., Pizzighella, S., Mazzi, R., Solbiati, M., Concia, A., & Bassetti, D. (1989). Nosocomial epidemic of active tuberculosis among HIV-infected patients. *Lancet, 2,* 1502–1504.

Dodd, C. L., Greenspan, D., & Greenspan, J. S. (1991). Oral Kaposi's sarcoma in a woman as a first indication of HIV infection. *Journal of the American Dental Association, 122,* 61–63.

Dragic, T., Litwin, V., Allaway, G. P., Martin, S. R., Huang, Y., Nagashima, K. A., Cayanan, C., Maddon, P. J., Koup, R. A., Moore, J. P., & Paxton, W. A. (1996). HIV-1 entry into CD4+ cells is mediated by the chemokine receptor CC-CKR-5. *Nature, 381,* 667–673.

Duma, R. J. (1992) Pneumococcal pneumonia. In Wyngaarden, J. B., Smith, L. H., & Bennett, L. C. (Eds.), *Cecil textbook of medicine: Vol. 2.* (19th ed., pp. 1608–1615). Philadelphia, PA: W. B. Saunders Company.

Emery, L. J., Anderson, G. R., & Annin, J. B. (1992). Child welfare concerns. In A. C. Crocker, H. J. Cohen, & T. A. Kastner (Eds.), *HIV infection and developmental disabilities: A resource for service providers* (pp. 95–103). Baltimore, MD: Paul H. Brookes.

Engstrom, J. W., Lowenstein, D. H., & Bredesen, D. E. (1989). Cerebral infarctions and transient neurologic deficits associated with AIDS. *American Journal of Medicine, 86*(5), 528–532.

Epstein, L. G., Sharer, L. R., Joshi, V. V., Jojas, M. M., Koenigsberger, M. R., & Oleske, J. M. (1985). Progressive encephalopathy in children with acquired immune deficiency syndrome. *Annals of Neurology, 17,* 488–496.

Eyster, E. M., Goedert, J. J., Sarngadharan, M. G., Weiss, S. H., Gallo, R. C., & Blattner, W. A. (1985). Development and early natural history of HTLV-III antibodies in persons with hemophilia. *Journal of the American Medical Association (JAMA), 253,* 2219–2223.

Fahey, J. L., Talyor, J. M. G., Deetels, R., Hofmann, B., Melmed, R., Nishanian, P., & Giorgi, J. V. (1990). The prognostic value of cellular and serotologic markers in infection with human immunodeficiency virus type 1. *New England Journal of Medicine, 322*(3), 166–172.

Faulstich, M. (1986). Acquired immune deficiency syndrome: An overview of central nervous system complications and neuropsychological sequelae. *International Journal of Neuroscience, 30,* 249–254.

Feng, Y., Broder, C. C., Kennedy, P. E., & Berger, E A. (1996). HIV-1 entry cofactor: Functional cDNA cloning of a sevin-transmembrane, G protein-coupled receptor. *Science, 272,* 872–877.

Fischl, M. A., Richman, D. D., Grieco, M. H., Gottlieb, M. S., Volberding, P. A., Laskin, L., Leedom, J. M., Groopman, J. E., Mildvan, D., Schooley, R. T., Jackson, G. G., Durack, D. T., King, D., & the AZT Collaborative Working Group. (1987). The efficacy of azidothymidine (AZT) and the treatment of patients with AIDS and the AIDS-related complex. A double-blind placebo controlled trial. *New England Journal of Medicine, 317*(4), 185–191.

Flower, W. M. & Sooy, C. D. (1987). AIDS: An introduction for speech-language pathologists and audiologists. *Asha, 29*(11), 25–30.

Friedman, S. L. (1994). Dysphagia and odynophagia due to esophagitis. In P. T. Cohen, M. A. Sande, & P. A. Volberding (Eds.), *The AIDS knowledge base* (2nd ed., pp. 5.21-1– 5.21-6). Waltham, MA: The Medical Publishing Group.

FDA Public Health Advisory. (1997, June). Reports of diabetes and hyperglycemia in patients receiving protease inhibitors for the treatment of human immunodeficiency virus (HIV).

Gallo, R. C., Salahuddin, S. Z., Popovic, M., Shearer, G. M., Kaplan, M., Haynes, B. F., Palker, T. J., Redfield, R., Oleske, J., Safai, B., White, G., Foster, P., & Markham, P. D. (1984). Frequent detection and isolation of cytopathic retroviruses (HTLV-III) from patients with AIDS and at risk for AIDS. *Science, 224,* 500–503.

Gay, L. R. (1996). *Educational research: Competencies for analysis and application* (5th ed.). Englewood Cliffs, NJ: Prentice Hall.

Gerberding, J. L. (1995). Management of occupational exposures to bloodborne viruses. *New England Journal of Medicine, 332*(7), 444–451.

Gherman, C. R., Ward, R. R., & Bassis, M. L. (1988). *Pneumocystis carinii* otitis media and mastoiditis as the initial manifestation of the acquired immunodeficiency syndrome. *American Journal of Medicine, 85,* 250–252.

Goldfarb, J. (1993). Breast feeding: AIDS and other infectious disease. *Clinics of Perinatology, 20,* 225.

Gordon, S. M., Eaton, M. E., George, R., Larsen, S., Lukehart, S. A., Kuypers, J., Marra, C. M., & Thompson, S. (1994). The response of symptomatic neurosyphilis to highdose intravenous penicillin G in patients with human immunodeficiency virus infection. *New England Journal of Medicine, 331*(22), 1469–1473.

Gray, F., Hurtrel, M., & Hurtrel, B. (1993). Annotation. Early central nervous system changes in human immunodeficiency virus (HIV)-infection. *Neuropathology & Applied Neurobiology, 19*(1), 3–9.

Greenspan, D., Greenspan, J. S., Pindborg, J. J., & Schiodt, M. (1990). *AIDS and the mouth.* Copenhagen: Munkgaard.

Greenspan, J. S., & Greenspan, D. (1995). Oral complications of HIV infection. In M. A. Sande & P. A. Volberding (Eds.), *The Medical Management of AIDS.* (4th ed., pp. 224–240). Philadelphia, PA: W. B. Saunders.

Greenwood, D. U. (1991). Neuropsychological aspects of AIDS dementia complex: What clinicians need to know. *Professional Psychology: Research and Practice, 22*(5), 407–409.

Griffith, B. P., & Booss, J. (1994). Neurologic infections of the fetus and newborn. *Neurologic Clinics, 12*(3), 541–564.

Groopman, J. E., Salahuddin, S. Z., Sarngadharan, M. G., Markham, P. D., Gonda, M., Sliski, A., & Gallo, R. C. (1984). HTLV-III in saliva of people with AIDS-related complex and healthy homosexual men at risk for AIDS. *Science, 226,* 447–449.

Grossman, M. (1995). Pediatric AIDS. In M. A. Sande & P. A. Volberding (Eds.), *The Medical Management of AIDS* (4th ed., pp. 632–647). Philadelphia, PA: W. B. Saunders.

Haddad, J., Brager, R., Bluestone, C. D. (1992). Infections of the ears, nose and throat in children with primary immunodeficiencies. *Archives of Otolaryngology and Head and Neck Surgery, 118,* 138–141.

Hart, C. W., Cokely, C. G., Schupbach, J., Dal Canto, M., & Coppelson, W. (1989). Neurotologic findings of a patient with acquired immune deficiency syndrome. *Ear and Hearing, 10,* 68–76.

Heaton, R. K., Velin, R. A., McCutchan, A., Gulevich, S. J., Atkinson, J. H., Wallace, M. R., Godfrey, H. P. D., Kirson, D. A., Grant, I. & The HNRC Group. (1994). Neuropsychological impairment in human immunodeficiency virus-infection: Implications for employment. *Psychosomatic Medicine, 56*(1), 8–17.

Heffernan, J. J., Osten, C. M., & Dunn, E. (1993). Weight loss and malnutrition. In H. Libman & R. A. Witzburg (Eds.), *HIV infection: A clinical manual* (2nd ed., pp. 65–73). Boston, MA: Little, Brown and Company.

Hengel, R. L., Watts, N. B., & Lennox, J. L. (1997). Benign symmetric lipomatosis associated with protease inhibitors. *Lancet, 350,* 1596.

Hickey, M. S., & Weaver, K. E. (1988). Nutritional management of patients with ARC and AIDS. *Gastroenterology Clinics of North America, 17,* 545–561.

Ho, D. D., Schooley, R. T., Rota, T. R., Kaplan, J. C., Flynn, T., Salahuddin, S. Z., Gonda, M. A., & Hirsch, M. S. (1984). HTLV-III in the semen and blood of a healthy homosexual man. *Science, 226,* 451–453.

Ho, D. D., Rota, T. R., Schooley, R. T., Kaplan, J. C., Allan, J. D., Groopman, J. E., Resnick, L., Felsenstein D., Andrews, C. A. & Hirsch, M. S. (1985). Isolation of HTLV-III from cerebrospinal fluid and neural tissues of patients with neurologic syndromes related to the acquired immunodeficiency syndrome. *New England Journal of Medicine, 313*(24), 1493–1497.

Ho, D. D., Pomerantz, R. J., & Kaplan, J. C. (1987). Pathogenesis of infection with human immunodeficiency virus. *New England Journal of Medicine, 317*(5), 278–286.

Holland, J. C. & Tross, S. (1985). The psychosocial and neuropsychiatric sequelae of the acquired immunodeficiency syndrome and related disorders. *Annals of Internal Medicine, 103*(5), 760–764.

Hollander, H., & Stringari, S. (1987). Human immunodeficiency virus-associated meningitis: Clinical course and correlations. *American Journal of Medicine, 83*(5), 813–816.

Hoover, D. R., Saah, A. J., Bacellar, H., Phair, J., Detels, R., Anderson, R., & Kaslow, R. A., for the Multicenter AIDS Cohort Study. (1993). Clinical manifestations of AIDS of the era of *Pneumocystis* prophylaxis. *New England Journal of Medicine, 329*(26), 1922–1926.

Hopkins, K. M. (1989). Emerging patterns of services and case finding for children with HIV infection. *Mental Retardation, 27,* 219–222.

Jacobs, J. L., Libby, D. M., Winters, R. A., Gelmont, D. M., Fried, E. D., Hartman, B. J., & Laurence, J. (1991). *Pneumocystis carinii* pneumonia in adults without predisposing illnesses. *New England Journal of Medicine, 324*(4), 246–250.

Jacobson, M. A. (1995). Disseminated Mycobacterium avium complex and other bacterial infections. In M. A. Sande & P. A. Volberding (Eds.), *The Medical Management of AIDS* (4th ed., pp. 402–415). Philadelphia, PA: W. B. Saunders.

Jansen, J. (1995). Pediatric AIDS Foundation: National Registry of Pediatric Long Term Survivors, First Year Summary.

Jenkins, M. (1996). Human immunodeficiency virus Type 1 infection in infants and children. In A. M. Rudolf (Ed.), *Rudolf's pediatrics* (20th ed., pp. 655–661). Stamford, CT: Appleton and Lange.

Jones, D., & Molaghan, J. B. (1995). HIV nursing care. In M. A. Sande & P. A. Volberding (Eds.), *The Medical Management of AIDS* (4th ed., pp. 680–695). Philadelphia, PA: W. B. Saunders.

Kastner, T., & Friedman, D. (1988). Pediatric acquired immune deficiency syndrome and the prevention of mental retardation. *Developmental and Behavioral Pediatrics, 9,* 47–48.

Kieburtz, K. D., Eskin, T. A., Ketonen, L., & Tuite, M. J. (1993). Opportunistic cerebral vasculopathy and stroke in patients with the acquired immunodeficiency syndrome. *Archives of Neurology, 50*(4), 430–432.

Kieburtz, K., Ketonen, L., Cox, C., Grossman, H., Holloway, R., Booth, H., Hickey, C., Feigin, A., & Caine, E. D. (1996). Cognitive performance and regional brain volume in human immunodeficiency virus type 1 infection. *Archives of Neurology, 53*(2), 155–158.

Kirk, J., & Miller, M. (1986). *Reliability, validity and qualitative research.* Beverly Hills, CA: Sage.

Klatzmann, D., Champagne, E., Chamaret, S., Gruest, J., Guetard, D., Hercend, T., Gluckman, J-C., & Montagnier, L. (1984). T-lymphocyte T4 molecule behaves as the receptor for human retrovirus LAV. *Nature, 312,* 767–768.

Kletter, R., Jeremy, R. J., Rumsey, C., Weintraub, P., & Cowan, M. (1989). A prospective study of the mental and motor development of infants born to HIV infected intravenous drug abusing mothers. *V International Conference on AIDS: Abstracts 5,* 225.

Kohan, D., Hammerschlag, P. E., & Holiday, R. A. (1990). Otologic disease in AIDS patients: CT correlation. *Laryngoscope, 100,* 1326–1330.

Kotler, D. P., Wang, J., & Pierson, R. N. (1985). Body composition studies in patients with the acquired immunodeficiency syndrome. *American Journal of Clinical Nutrition, 42,* 1255–1265.

Kovacs, A., Leaf, H. L., & Simberkoff, M. S. (1997). Bacterial infections. *Medical Clinics of North America, 81*(2), 319–343.

Kozlowski, P. (1992). Neuropathology of HIV infection in children. In A. C. Crocker, H. J. Cohen, & T. A. Kastner (Eds.), *HIV infection and developmental disabilities: A resource for service providers* (pp. 25–32). Baltimore, MD: Paul H. Brookes.

Krasinski, K., Borkowsky, W., & Holzman, R. S. (1989). Prognosis of human immunodeficiency virus infection in children and adolescents. *Pediatric Infectious Disease Journal, 8,* 216–220.

Kwartler, J. A., Linthicum, F. H., Jahn, A. F., & Hawke, M. (1991). Sudden hearing loss due to AIDS-related cryptococcal meningitis: A temporal bone study. *Otolaryngology—Head and Neck Surgery, 104*(2), 265–269.

Lalwani, A. K., & Sooy, C. D. (1992). Otologic and neurotologic manifestations of acquired immunodeficiency syndrome. *Otolarynogologic Clinics of North America, 25*(6), 1183–1197.

Larsen, C. R. (1996). *Associated Communication Disorders and Dysphagia in Adults with HIV-1 and Secondary CNS Lesions.* Unpublished master's independent study, University of North Dakota, Grand Forks.

Levy, J. A., Kaminsky, L. S., Morrow, W. J. W. Steimer, K., Luciw, P., Dina, D., Hoxie, J., & Ashiro L. (1985). Infection by the retrovirus associated with the acquired immunodeficiency. *Annals of Internal Medicine, 103*(5), 694–699

Levy, R. M., Bredesen, D. E., & Rosenblum, M. L. (1985). Neurological manifestations of the acquired immunodeficiency syndrome (AIDS): Experience at UCSF and review of the literature. *Journal of Neurosurgery, 62*(4), 475–495.

Levy, R. M., Bredesen, D. E., Rosenblum, M. L., & Davis, R. L. (1989). Central nervous system dysfunction in AIDS. In J. A. Levy (Ed.). *AIDS pathogenesis and treatment* (pp. 368–401). New York: Marcel Dekker, Inc.

Levy, R. M. & Berger, J. R. (1992). Neurologic complications of HIV infection: diagnosis, therapy, and functional considerations. In J. Mukand (Ed.), *Rehabilitation for patients with HIV disease* (pp. 55–76). New York: McGraw-Hill, Inc.

Lewis, J. L., & Rabinovich, S. (1972). The wide spectrum of cryptococcal infections. *American Journal of Medicine, 53*(3), 315–321.

Lifschitz, M., Hanson, C., Wilson, G., & Shearer, W. T. (1989). Behavioral changes in children with human immunodeficiency virus (HIV) infection. *V International Conference on AIDS: Abstracts, 5,* 316.

Luban, J., Bossolt, K.L., Franke, E. K., Kalpana, G. V., & Goff, S. (1993). Human immunodeficiency virus type 1 virus gag protein binds to cyclophilins A and B. *Cell, 73*(6), 1067–1078.

Luft, B. J., Hafner, R., Korzun, A. H., Leport, C., Antoniskis, D., Bosler, E. M., Bourland, d. d., Uttamchandani, R., Fuhrer, J., Jacobson, J., Morlat, P., Vilde, J-L., Remington, J. S., & Members of the ACTG 077p/ANRSs Study Team. Toxoplasmic encephalitis in patients with the acquired immunodeficiency syndrome. *New England Journal of Medicine, 329*(14), 995–1000.

Maddon, P. J., Dagleish, A. G., McDougal, J. S., Clapham, P. R., Weiss, R. A., & Axel, R. (1986). The T4 cell encodes the AIDS virus receptor and is expressed in the immune system and the brain. *Cell, 47*(3), 333–348.

Madriz, J. J., & Herrera, G. (1995). Human immunodeficiency virus and acquired immune deficiency syndrome AIDS-related hearing disorders. *Journal of the American Academy of Audiology, 6,* 358–364.

Mann, J., Tarantola, D. J. M., Netter, T. W. (1992). *A global report: AIDS in the world.* Cambridge, MA: Harvard University Press.

Marcus, J. C., Butler, C. A., Hittleman, J. H., Mendez, H., Goedert, J. J., & Willoughby, A. (1989). Pattern of neurological abnormalities in infants at risk for developing AIDS. *V International Conference on AIDS: Abstracts, 5,* 316.

Marcusen, D. C., & Sooy, C. D. (1985). Otolaryngologic and head and neck manifestations of acquired immunodeficiency syndrome AIDS). *Laryngoscope, 95,* 401–405.

Marshall, C. & Rossman, G. B. (1995). *Designing qualitative research* (2nd ed.). Thousand Oaks, CA: Sage.

Maruff, P., Currie, J., Malone, V., McArthur-Jackson, c., Mulhall, B., & Benson, E. (1994). Neuropsychological characterization of the AIDS dementia complex and rationalization of a test battery. *Archives of Neurology, 51*(7), 689–695.

Marx, G. L. (1989). Wider use of AIDS drugs advocated. *Science, 245,* 8–11.

Masliah, E., Achim, C. L., Ge, N., DeTeresa, R., Terry, R. D., & Wiley, C. A. (1992). Spectrum of human immunodeficiency virus associated neocortical damage. *Annals of Neurology, 32*(3), 321–329.

McArthur, J. C., Cohen, B. A., Selnes, O. A., Kumar, A. J., Cooper, K., McArthur, J. H., Soucy, G., Cornblath, D. R., Chmiel, J. S., Wang, M-C., Starkey, D. L., Ginzburg, H., Ostrow, D. G., Johnson, R. T., Phair, J. P., & Polk, B. F. (1989). Low prevalence of neurological and neuropsychological abnormalities in otherwise healthy HIV-1 infected individuals: Results from the Multicenter AIDS Cohort Study. *Annals of Neurology, 26*(5), 601–611.

McGill, T. (1978). Mycotic infections of the temporal bone. *Archives of Otolaryngology, 104*(3), 104–144.

Mehta, P. & Kula, R. W. (1992). Neurologic manifestations of human immunodeficiency virus infection. *Otolaryngologic Clinics of North America, 25*(6), 1249–1286.

Mellors, J. W., Rinaldo, C. R., Gupta, P., White, R. M., Todd, J. A., & Kingsley, L. A. (1996). Prognosis in HIV-1 infection predicted by the quantity of virus in plasma. *Science, 272,* 1167–1170.

Meyaard, L., Otto, S. A., Keet, I. P. M., Ross, M. T. L., & Miedema, F. (1992). Programmed death of T cells in HIV-1 infection. *Science, 257,* 217–219.

Miles, M. S. & Huberman, A. M. (1984). *Qualitative data analysis: A sourcebook of new methods* (2nd ed.). Beverly Hills, CA: Sage.

Miller E. N., Selnes, O. A., McArthur, J. C., Satz, P., Becker, J. T., Cohen, B. A., Sheridan, K., Machado, A. M., Van Gorp, W. G., & Visscher, B. (1990). Neuropsychological performance in HIV-1–infected homosexual men: The multicenter AIDS cohort study (MACS). *Neurology, 40*(2), 197–203.

Miller, M. J., & Remington, J. S. (1991). Toxoplasmosis in infants and children with HIV infection or AIDS. In P. A. Pizzo & C. M. Wilfert (Eds.), *Pediatric AIDS: The challenge of HIV infection in infants, children and adolescents* (pp. 299–307). Baltimore: Williams & Wilkens.

Minkoff, H., Nanda, D., Menez, R., & Fikrig, S. (1987). Pregnancies resulting in infants with acquired immunodeficiency syndrome or AIDS-related complex: Follow-up of mothers, children, and subsequently born siblings. *Obstetrics and Gynecology, 69,* 288–291.

Moore, R. D., Keruly, J. C., Chaisson, R. E. (1997). *Effectiveness of combination antiretroviral therapy in clinical practice.* 37th Interscience Conference on Antimicrobial Agents and Chemotherapy (ICAAC), Toronto, Ontario, Canada, September 28–October 1, 1997, Abstract I-176.

Morris, M. S., & Prasad, S. (1990). Otologic disease in the acquired immunodeficiency syndrome. *Ear Nose Throat Journal, 69,* 451–453.

Moss, H., Wolters, P., Eddy, J., Weiner, L., Pizzo, P., & Brouwers, P. (1989). The effects of encephalopathy and AZT treatment on the social and emotional behavior in pediatric AIDS. *V International Conference on AIDS: Abstracts, 5,* 328.

Moss, H., Wolters, P., El-Amin, D., Butler, K., Brouwers, P., & Pizzo, P. (1990). The use of videotaped behavior samples of pediatric AIDS patients to evaluate psychosocial changes associated with encephalopathy before and after treatment. *VI International Conference on AIDS: Abstracts, 6,* 131.

Murray, A. B., Greenhouse, P. R. D. H., Nelson, W. L. C., Norman, J. E., Jeffries, D. J., & Anderson, J. (1991). Coincident acquisition of *Neisseria gonorrhea* and HIV from fellatio. *Lancet, 338,* 1088.

Navia, B. A., Jordan B. D., & Price, R. W. (1986). The AIDS dementia complex: I. Clinical features. *Annals of Neurology, 19*(6), 517–524.

Neuen-Jacob, E., Arendt, G., von Giesen, H. J., & Wechsler, W. (1996). Neuronal cell apoptosis in the basal ganglia occurs early in the course of HIV encephalitis and may precede the clinical signs of HIV-1 associated dementia. *Neuropathology & Applied Neurobiology, 22*(Suppl. 1), 16–17.

Nevell, N. J., Bewley, A. P., & Chopra, S. (1995). Bacillary angiomatosis with cutaneous and oral lesions in an HIV-infected patient from the U. K. *British Journal of Dermatology, 132,* 113.

Novick, B. E. (1989). Pediatric AIDS: A medical overview. In J. M. Seibert & R. A. Olson (Eds.), *Children, adolescents, and AIDS* (pp. 1–23). Lincoln: University of Nebraska Press.

Oleske, J. (1987). Natural history of HIV infection II. In B. K. Silverman & A. Waldell, (Eds.), *Surgeon general's workshop report on children with HIV infection* (pp. 73–84). Washington, DC: Health and Human Services Department.

Ollo, C., Johnson, R., & Graftman, J. (1991). Signs of cognitive changes in HIV disease: An event-related brain potential study. *Neurology, 41,* 209–215.

Osguthorpe, J. D. (1992). Occupational human immunodeficiency virus exposure. *Otolaryngologic Clinics of North America, 25*(6), 1341–1353.

O'Sullivan, P., Linke, R. A., & Dalton, S. (1985). Evaluation of body weight and nutritional status among AIDS patients. *Journal of the American Dietetic Association, 85,* 1483–1484.

Pang, S., Shlesinger, Y., Daar, E. S., Moudgil, T., Ho D. D., Chen, I. S. Y. (1992). Rapid generation of sequence variation during primary HIV-1 infection. *AIDS, 6,* 453–460.

Petito, C. K., Navia, B. A.., Cho, E-S, Jordan, B. D., George, D. C., & Price, R. W. (1985). Vacuolar myelopathy pathologically resembling subacute combined degeneration in patients with the acquired immunodeficiency syndrome. *New England Journal of Medicine, 312*(14), 874–879.

Petito, C. K., Cho, E-S., Lemann, W., Navia, B. A., & Price, R. W. (1986). Neuropathology of AIDS: An autopsy review. *Journal of Neuropathology and Experimental Neurology, 45*(6), 635–646.

Petito, C. K., Vecchio, D., & Chen, Y-T. (1994). HIV antigen and DNA in AIDS spinal cords correlate with macrophage infiltration but not with vacuolar myelopathy. *Journal of Neuropathology and Experimental Neurology, 53*(1), 86–94.

Phelan, J. A. (1997). Oral manifestations of human immunodeficiency virus infection. *Medical Clinics of North America, 81*(2), 511–530.

Piot, P. (1997). *Global epidemiology of HIV infection.* 37th Interscience Conference on Antimicrobial Agents and Chemotherapy (ICAAC), Toronto, Ontario, Canada, September 28–October 1, 1997, Abstract S-33.

Pizzo, P. A. (1990). Pediatric AIDS: Problems with problems. *Journal of Infectious Diseases, 161,* 316–325.

Popovic, M., Sarngadharan, M. G., Read, E., & Gallo, R. C. (1984). Detection, isolation, and continuous production of cytopathic retroviruses (HTLV-III). *Science, 224,* 497–500.

Porter, S. B., & Sande, M. A. (1992). Toxoplasmosis of the central nervous system in the acquired immunodeficiency syndrome. *New England Journal of Medicine, 327*(23), 1643–1648.

Pressman, H. (1992). Communication disorders and dysphagia in pediatric AIDS. *ASHA, 34,* 45–47.

Pressman, H., & Morrison, S. H. (1988). Dysphagia in the pediatric AIDS population. *Dysphagia, 2,* 166–169.

Price, R. W., Brew, B., Sidtis, J., Rosenblum, M., Scheck, A. C. & Cleary, P. (1988). The brain in AIDS: Central nervous system HIV-1 infection and AIDS dementia complex. *Science, 239,* 586–592.

Price, R. W., Brew, B. J., & Roke, M. (1992). Central and peripheral nervous system complications of HIV-1 infection and AIDS. In T. Vincent, J., Jr., Hellman, S., & Rosenberg, S. A. (Eds.). (1992). *AIDS: Etiology, diagnosis, treatment, and prevention* (3rd ed., pp. 237–257). Philadelphia, PA: J. B. Lippincott

Principi, N., Marchisio, P., Tornaghi, R., Ornato, J., Massinori, E., & Picco, P. (1991). Acute otitis media in human immunodeficiency virus-infected children. *Pediatrics, 88,* 566–571.

Rabeneck, L., Popovic, M., Gartner, S., McLean, D. M., McLeod, W. A., Read, E., Wong, K. K., & Boyko, W. J. (1990). Acute HIV infection presenting with painful swallowing and esophageal ulcers. *Journal of the American Medical Association (JAMA), 263*(17), 2318–2322.

Ratner, L., Haseltine, W., Patarca, R., Livak, K. J., Starcich, B., Josephs, S. F., Doran, E. R., Rafalski, A., Whitehorn, E. A., Baumeister, K., Invanoff, L., Petteway, S. R., Jr., Pearson, K. L., Lautenberger, J. A., Papas, T. S., Ghrayeb, J., Chang, N. T., Gallo, R. C., & Wong-Stall, F. (1985). Complete nucleotide sequence of the AIDS virus HTLV-III. *Nature, 313,* 277–284.

Raufman, J. P. (1988). Odynophagia/dysphagia in AIDS. *Gastroenterologic Clinics of North America, 17*(3), 599–614.

Resnick, L., diMarzo-Veronese, F., Schupach, J., Tourtellotte, W. W., Ho, D.D, Muller, F., Shaphak, P., Vogt, M., Groopman, J. E., Markham, P. D., & Gallo, R. C. (1985). Intra-blood-brain-barrier synthesis of HTLV-III- specific IgG in patients with neurologic symptoms associated with AIDS or AIDS related complex. *New England Journal of Medicine, 313*(24), 1498–1504

Respler, D. S., & Karas, D. E. (1996). Otolaryngologic manifestations of HIV infection in children. In C. D. Bluestone, S. E. Stool, & M. A. Kenna (Eds.), *Pediatric otolaryngology* (3rd ed., Vol. 1, pp. 99–112). Philadelphia: W. B. Saunders.

Ruane, P. J. (1997). *Atypical accumulations of fatty tissue.* 37th Interscience Conference on Antimicrobial Agents and Chemotherapy (ICAAC), Toronto, Ontario, Canada, September 28–October 1, 1997, Abstract I-185.

Rubin, J. S., & Honigsberg, R. (1990). Sinusitis in patients with the acquired immunodeficiency syndrome. *Ear Nose Throat Journal, 69,* 460–4463.

Saag, M. S. (1992). Prevention of HIV Infection. In Wyngaarden, J. B., Smith, L. H., & Bennett, L. C. (Eds.), *Cecil Textbook of Medicine: Vol. 2.* (19th ed., pp. 1925–1928). Philadelphia, PA: W. B. Saunders Company.

Sahakian, B.J., Elliot, R., Low, N., Mehta, M., Clark, R. T. & Pozniak, A. L. (1995). Neuropsychological deficits in tests of executive function in asymptomatic and symptomatic HIV-1 seropositive men. *Psychological Medicine. 25*(4), 1233–1246.

Schneider, W. D., Simpson, D. M., Nielson, S., Gold, J. W. M., Metroka, C. E., & Posner, J. B. (1983). Neurological complications of acquired immune deficiency syndrome: Analysis of 50 patients. *Annals of Neurology, 14*(4), 403–418.

Schiodt, M., & Pindborg, J. J. (1987). AIDS and the oral cavity. Epidemiology and clinical oral manifestations of human immune deficiency virus infection: A review. *International Journal of Oral Maxillofacial Surgery, 16,* 1.

Scott, G. B., Hutto, C., Makuch, R. W., Mastrucci, M. T., O'Connor, T., Mitchell, C. D., Trapido, E. J., & Parks, W. P. (1989). Survival in children with perinatally acquired human immunodeficiency virus Type 1 infection. *New England Journal of Medicine, 321,* 1791–1796.

Seidel, J. F. (1991). The development of a comprehensive pediatric HIV developmental service program. In A. Rudigier (Ed.), *Technical report on developmental disabilities and HIV Infection (No. 7)* (pp. 1–4). Silver Spring, MD: American Association of University Affiliated Programs.

Seidel, J. F., & Seibert, J. M. (1990). *Pediatric HIV infection: Guidelines for psychosocial case management.* Unpublished manuscript, University of Miami School of Medicine, Miami, FL.

Sepkowitz, K. A. (1996). Occupationally acquired infections in health care workers: Part I. *Annals of Internal Medicine, 125,* 826.

Shaw, G. M., Hahn, B. H., Arya, S. K., Groopman, J. E., Gallo, R. C., & Wong-Staal, F. (1984). Molecular characterization of human T-cell leukemia (lymphotropic) virus type III in the acquired immune deficiency syndrome. *Science, 226*(4679), 1165–1171.

Shor-Posner, G., Morgan, R., Wilkie, F., Eisdorfer, C., & Baum, M. K. (1995). Plasma cobalamin levels affect information processing speed in a longitudinal study of HIV-1 disease. *Archives of Neurology, 52*(2), 195–198.

Siliciano, R. (1997). *Latent reservoir of HIV.* 37th Interscience Conference on Antimicrobial Agents and Chemotherapy (ICAAC), Toronto, Ontario, Canada, September 28–October 1, 1997, Abstract S-36.

Simpson, D. M., & Berger, J. R. (1996). Neurologic manifestation of HIV infection. *Medical Clinics of North America, 80*(6), 1363–1394.

Smith, M. E., & Canalis, R. F. (1989). Otologic manifestation of AIDS: The otosyphilis connection. *Laryngoscope, 99*(4), 365–372.

Solorio, M. R., & Stevens, N. G. (1997). Health care of the adolescent. In R. B. Taylor (Ed.), *Family medicine: Principles and practice* (5th ed., pp. 207–218). New York: Springer.

Sooy, C. D. (1987). The impact of AIDS on otolaryngology—head and neck surgery. In N. Myers (Ed). *Advances in otolaryngology—head and neck surgery* (Vol. 1, pp. 1–27). Chicago, IL: Year Book Medical Publishers.

Stern, R. A., Silva, S. G., Chaisoon, N., & Evans, D. l. (1996). Influence of cognitive reserve on neuropsychological functioning in asymptomatic human immunodeficiency virus-1 infection. *Archives of Neurology, 53*(2), 148–153.

Stout, J. C., Salmon, D. P., Butters, M., Peavy, G.., Heindel, W. C., Delis, D. C., Ryan, L., Atkinson, J. H., Chandler, J. l., Grant, I. & The HNRC Group. (1995). Decline in working memory associated with HIV infection. *Psychological Medicine, 25*(4), 1221–1232.

Straus, D. J. (1997). Human immunodeficiency virus-associated lymphomas. *Medical Clinics of North America, 81*(2), 495–510.

Swales, T. P. (1991). *Cognitive and developmental evaluation of perinatal HIV-1 infection during infancy.* Unpublished doctoral dissertation, University of Miami, Coral Gables, FL.

Tami, T. A., & Wawrose, S F. (1992). Diseases of the nose and paranasal sinuses in the human immunodeficiency virus-infected population. *Otolaryngologic Clinics of North America, 25*(6), 1199–1210.

Tanowitz, H. B., Simon, D., Weiss, L. M., Noyer, C., Coyle, C., & Wittner, M. (1996). Gastrointestinal manifestations. *Medical Clinics of North America, 80*(6), 1395–1414.

Tay-Kearney, M-L., & Jabs, D. A. (1996). Ophthalmic complications of HIV infections. *Medical Clinics of North America, 80*(6), 1471–1483.

Thompson, C., Salvato, P., Stroud, S., & Hasheeve, D. (1993). Etiology of acute sinusitis in HIV infection (Abstract WS-B08–6). IX International Conference on AIDS, Berlin, Germany.

Tramontana, M. C., & Hooper, S. R. (1989). Neuropsychology of child psychopathology. In C. R. Reynolds & E. Fletcher-Janzen (Eds.), *Handbook of clinical child neuropsychology* (pp. 87–106). New York: Plenum Press.

Vincent, T., DeVita, J., Jr., Hellman, S., & Rosenberg, S. T. (Eds.). (1992). *AIDS: Etiology, diagnosis, treatment and prevention* (3rd ed.). Philadelphia, PA: J. B. Lippincott Company.

Vidmar, L., Poljak, M., Tomazic, J., Seme, K., & Klavs, I. (1996). Transmission of HIV-1 by human bite. *Lancet, 347,* 1762–1763.

Vinters, H. V., & Anders, K. H. (1990). *Neuropathology of AIDS.* Boca Raton, FL: CRC Press.

Volberding, P. A., Lagakos, S. W., Koch, M. A., Pettinelli, C., Myers, M. W., Booth, D. K., Balfour, H. H., Reichman, R. C., Bartlett, J. A., Hirsch, M. S., Murphy, R. L., Hardy, W. D., Soeiro, R., Fischl, M. A., Bartlett, J. G., Merigan, T. C., Hyslop, N. E., Richman D. D., Valentine, F. T., Corey, L., & the AIDS Clinical Trials Group of the National Institute of Allergy and Infectious Diseases. (1990). Zidovudine in asymptomatic human immunodeficiency virus infection: A controlled trial in persons with fewer than 500 CD4-positive cells per cubic millimeter. *New England Journal of Medicine, 322*(14), 941–949.

Walker, B. D. (1992). Immunology related to AIDS. In Wyngaarden, J. B., Smith, L. H., & Bennett, L. C. (Eds.), *Cecil textbook of medicine: Vol. 2.* (19th ed., pp. 1908–1912). Philadelphia, PA: W. B. Saunder Company.

Walsh, T. J., & Butler, K. M. (1991). Fungal infections complicating pediatric AIDS. In P. A. Pizzo & C. M. Wilfert (Eds.), *Pediatric AIDS: The challenge of HIV infection in infants, children and adolescents* (pp. 299–307). Baltimore: Williams & Wilkens.

Walzer, P. D. (1991). *Pneumocystis carinii*—new clinical spectrum? *New England Journal of Medicine, 321*(4), 1476.

Wara, D. W., & Dorenbaum, A. (1995). Pediatric AIDS: Perinatal transmission and early diagnosis. In M. A. Sande & P. A. Volberding (Eds.), *The Medical Management of AIDS* (4th ed., pp. 626–631). Philadelphia, PA: W. B. Saunders.

Watkins, B. A., Dorn, H. H., Kelly, W. B., Armstrong, R. C., Potts, B. J., Michaels, F., Kufta, C.V. & Dubois-Dalcq, M. (1990). Specific tropism of HIV-1 for microglial cells in primary human brain cultures. *Science, 249,* 549–553.

Weiss, S. H. (1997). Risks and issues for the health care worker in the human immunodeficiency virus era. *Medical Clinics of North America, 81*(2), 555–575.

Welkoborsky, H. J., & Lowitzsch, K. (1992). Auditory brain stem responses in patients with human immunotropic virus infection of different stages. *Ear and Hearing, 13,* 55–57.

Wilcox, C. M. (1992). Esophageal disease in the acquired immunodeficiency syndrome: Etiology, diagnosis, and management. *American Journal of Medicine, 92*(4), 412–421.

Wilcox, C. M., Zaki, S. R., & Coffield, L. M. (1993). Localization of human immunodeficiency virus (HIV-1) by in-situ hybridization in esophageal ulcers: Further evidence refuting HIV as an esophageal pathogen. *Gastroenterology, 104,* A801.

Wilson, W. R. (1986). The relationship of the herpes virus to sudden hearing loss: A prospective clinical study and literature review. *Laryngoscope, 96,* 870–877.

Wiznia, A. A., Lambert, G., & Pavlakis, S. (1996). Pediatric HIV infection. *Medical Clinics of North America, 80*(6), 1309–1336.

Wolinsky, S. M., Wike, C. M., Korber, B. T. M., Hutto, C., Parks, W. P., Rosenblum, L. L., Kunstman, K. L., Furtado, M. R., & Munoz, J. L. (1992). Selective transmission of human immunodeficiency virus Type-1 variants from mothers to infants. *Science, 255,* 1134–1137.

World Health Organization (WHO). (1992). *Global programme on AIDS: Current and future dimensions of the HIV/AIDS pandemic. A capsule summary.* Geneva: WHO.

Wong-Staal, F., Shaw, G. M., Hahn, B. H., Salhuddin, S. Z., Popovic, M., Markham, P., Redfield, R., & Gallo, R. C. (1985). Genomic diversity of human T-lymphotropic virus type III (HTLV-III). *Science, 229,* 759–762.

Worley, J. M. & Price, R. W. (1992). Management of neurologic complications of HIV-1 infection and AIDS. In M. A. Sande & P. A. Volberding (Eds.), *The medical management of AIDS* (3rd ed., pp. 193–233). Philadelphia: W. B. Saunders Company.

Zagury, D., Bernard, J., Leibowitch, J., Safai, B., Groopman, J. E., Feldman, M., Sarngadharan, M. G., & Gallo, R. C. (1984). HTLV-III in cells cultured from the semen of two patients with AIDS. *Science, 226,* 449–451.

Zurlo, J. J., Feuerstein, I. M., Lebovics, R., & Lane, H. C. (1992). Sinusitis in HIV-1 infection. *American Journal of Medicine, 93,* 157–162.

Index